Contents

Foreword

I have been a trainer since 1976 and seen so many teaching aids come and go, just occasionally something really focused and useful comes along; *The Study Guide for General Practice Training* is such a tool. This book is an aid to learning that is of its time, authoritative, expert, clear and perhaps its greatest strength, demystifying of modern learning and assessment methods.

General practice may be the most difficult of all the medical disciplines to do really well. The knowing and the doing are difficult enough, but it is the synthesising, the sorting the wheat from the chaff, and the continuous learning from both patients and academia that are the really hard parts. On top of this, the ability to communicate well with patients, partners, consultants and primary care trusts is essential and not easy to learn, but using this guide with your trainer will give you a firm foundation to help you build a successful and fulfilling career.

The *Study Guide* has done a lot of the drudgery for you, you will know where to find things and there are ready made reading lists, but what I really hope is that the guide will fire your enthusiasm for general practice and make your passage through training just that bit more enjoyable.

Peter Tate
Convener of the Panel of Examiners of the
Royal College of Gencral Practitioners
March 2003

About the authors

Tim Swanwick is a Director of Postgraduate General Practice Education in the London Deanery.

Nav Chana is an Associate Director of Postgraduate General Practice Education in the London Deanery.

Both are practising general practitioners, examiners for the Royal College of General Practitioners and both have a wide experience of all aspects of general practice training and education.

Acknowledgements

We would like to acknowledge the hard work of colleagues in the former North East Thames Deanery who produced earlier editions of a *Study Guide for GP Registars* on which this book is based. We would also like to acknowledge the work of David Sales and the Syllabus Development Group of the Royal College of General Practitioners whose thoughts have informed some of the topic areas. Thank you.

1

The study guide and general practice training

Introduction

The *Study Guide* has been written to provide a specific aid to learning for the general practice (GP) registrar. Despite this focus, we hope that all learners in general practice, whether undertaking clinical attachments, returning to general practice after a career break, or simply wishing to refresh their professional knowledge, will find the book useful. The guide illustrates the range of topics that should be covered during GP training and indicates how best individual subjects might be approached.

Each GP learner will bring to the training period a different set of knowledge, skills and attitudes, depending on the hospital and general practice experience he, or she, has already obtained. The guide therefore begins with a section on the assessment of learning needs, needs that will vary enormously from learner to learner and, for the individual, throughout the course of training. Chapter 3 outlines the two end-point assessments that currently operate in GP training – summative assessment (SA) and the membership examination of the Royal College of General Practitioners (MRCGP).

We have also included two chapters on the process of learning. Chapter 4 focuses on important strands of educational theory that relate to adult learning, and outlines what might be expected during GP training. Chapter 5 discusses continuing professional development, and provides practical advice on putting together a personal learning, or personal development, plan.

The scope of general practice is so huge and all-embracing that a comprehensive guide is unrealistic, if not impossible. At the moment GP training lacks an explicit curriculum, although the soon to be published syllabus for the MRCGP examination[1] comes pretty close. When a curriculum finally does emerge, it is likely to be in the form of a competency framework built on the foundation stone of the General Medical Council's *Good Medical Practice*,[2] a document that has already been adapted for general practice by the Royal College of General Practitioners (RCGP).[3] The concept of a 'national curriculum' though comes with a health warning, and perhaps a more important outcome of training than the achievement of a completed checklist of professional competences, is that GP learners will have developed the ability to take into their subsequent careers an enthusiasm and commitment to continue self-development. We hope that this guide will start you on that journey.

How to use the guide

Chapter 6 of the guide is divided into topic areas. For each topic there is a set of objectives, 'What should be learned', and some suggestions for reaching those objectives, 'How to do it'. You and your trainer should identify many more learning opportunities than those mentioned here. The more unconventional they are the better. Learning should be fun.

- Look at the learning objectives. See if you and your trainer can write others.

- Try and uncover your own current learning needs. But beware: it is sometimes difficult to be honest or objective when analysing our own deficiencies. Discuss the best ways of doing this with your trainer who should have access to, or some ideas about a number of formative assessment tools. Several of these are outlined in Chapter 2.
- When you think you know what you need to learn, choose your learning methods. Those suggested in these notes may, or may not, suit you. Draw up a personal development plan (PDP). Practical advice for doing so is to be found in Chapter 5, but again your trainer should be able to help you.
- When you have tackled your chosen subject with the appropriate learning method, it is important to ascertain whether you have learned effectively. This will require further assessment. Look at some of the self-assessment problems in the guide. Are you confident that you can cope with them? Discuss issues that arise with your trainer.
- Each section of the guide includes a reading list of books and websites which recent registrars in our own deanery (London) have found helpful. The list is by no means exhaustive and your colleagues and peers will also have useful suggestions for essential reading.

As your training year progresses, your learning needs will develop and we hope that this book will become redundant. It helps though, to know where to start!

Study leave and courses

Study leave is granted under the terms of the registrar–trainer contract. A minimum allowance of 30 days per annum is specified by the Joint Committee of Postgraduate Training for General Practice to include attendance at the half-day release courses. Many deaneries specify a maximum study allowance, others don't, and you should discuss local arrangements with your trainer. In London, deanery policy is circulated to all trainers in a comprehensive *Trainer's Guide*.

You will receive, or be entitled to claim, a registrar allowance for course fees, travel and subsistence. Again, arrangements and amounts vary across the country and your local Department of Postgraduate General Practice will be able to advise you on your entitlement. Whatever it is, it won't be enough, so you will need to consider very carefully the courses that you intend to attend.

Who to contact with educational problems

We hope that your training year will run smoothly, but it is a time of transition and turbulence and occasionally, difficulties will arise. If you experience any particular educational problems, there are a number of people who may be able to help. Your trainer or local vocational training course organiser should be able to meet most of your needs but in the event of problematic issues which cannot be resolved at a local level, you should contact the Associate Dean (or Associate Director) for Postgraduate General Practice covering your area. The contact details for your area Associate Dean can be obtained from the administrators in your Department of Postgraduate General Practice.

References

1   Royal College of General Practitioners *A Syllabus for the MRCGP Examination*. (In preparation).

2   General Medical Council (2001) *Good Medical Practice* (3e). GMC, London.

3   Royal College of General Practitioners (RCGP) and General Practitioners Committee (GPC) (2002) *Good Medical Practice for General Practitioners*. RCGP, London.

2

Identifying your learning needs

How do I know what I don't know?

Before you start planning your learning programme, your own particular learning needs should be identified, a process that will require some honest reflection and self-assessment. There is plenty of evidence that we are not always very good at identifying our own educational needs and some structured ways of accomplishing this can be helpful. This process is called formative assessment. Formative assessment is purely educational and developmental and should not in any way be considered threatening or an imposition.

Formative assessment takes place during the course of teaching and is used to feedback into both teaching and learning. It is an ongoing process of uncovering where you are with a particular topic at a particular time and helping you find out what you need to know next. That is if you didn't know already.

Our various states of self-knowledge are succinctly summarised by the Johari window (*see* Figure 2.1).

The aim of the game is to expand the 'open' box at the expense of all others, i.e. it is best to know what you don't know, and for your trainer to be aware of those deficiencies, so that the two of you can work together on filling those gaps and planning your ongoing learning.

As the training year progresses, it is hoped that a relationship based on trust and openness develops between you and your

	Known to self	Unknown to self
Known to others	Open	Blind
Unknown to others	Hidden	Unknown

Figure 2.1: The Johari window.

trainer. In such an atmosphere, self disclosure is both possible and safe, and things in the 'hidden' box, i.e. those inadequacies known only to your self, can be brought out into the daylight and dealt with effectively. This is also the role of developmental appraisal.

More structured formative assessment tools may be useful for shrinking the 'blind' and 'unknown' boxes as they bring to your attention areas of ignorance that you never knew were there.

As enthusiasms come and go, you will need to balance satisfying your learning 'wants', those subjects which hold a particular fascination for you at a particular time, and learning 'needs', those areas that you need to address as a future general practitioner. Your trainer is there to help keep you on track.

Adults predominantly learn from experience. We also tend to learn best when we are experiencing some inadequacy in dealing with a particular life situation. General practice presents us with one life situation after another, providing a rich seam of learning needs to mine. There are various ways of tapping into and making the most of this experience and several such methods are outlined below.

As discussed earlier, sometimes more formal and objective methods of analysing our learning needs are required. There are many such assessment tools available ranging from multiple choice question papers to simulated surgeries and again, several of these are described. It is strongly encouraged that you keep a record of your learning needs as they are identified. Such a log could form a major part of your personal development plan (PDP).

Methods of learning needs analysis

Confidence rating scales

Confidence rating scales comprise of lists of topics covering the content of general practice. Registrars score themselves periodically through the year on the level of confidence reached in a particular subject. Such rating scales are useful at the outset of training to identify potentially weak areas but, as time goes on, our confidence in dealing with a particular problem may remain the same despite the acquisition of a considerable amount of knowledge and skill. The more we learn, the more we realise there is to learn!

There are many confidence rating scales available, e.g. The Wolverhampton Grid,[1] and your trainer's workshop or vocational training scheme may have developed its own.

Competence rating scales

Again, lists of topics are supplied but this time the trainer scores the registrar. The original vocational training rating scale was developed by the University of Manchester in 1976. This was replaced by a modified and shortened questionnaire in 1989.[2] As with all rating scales, they are somewhat tedious to complete and applying the results of such assessments can be a bruising experience unless handled sensitively by the trainer.

Learning needs generated by direct patient contact

Direct patient contact is by far the best way of generating learn-ing needs. The problem here though is avoiding being over-whelmed by a sense of inadequacy. Thirty plus patients a day are certainly capable of highlighting what you need to learn, the trick is to capture those needs as they arise and not let the moment pass without action.

A method of highlighting one's own educational needs in the surgery setting was developed by Dr Richard Eve and goes under the name of PUNs and DENs.[3] Dr Eve's idea was that many of our clinical encounters result in patients' needs not being met (Patients' Unmet Needs; PUNs). Some of these PUNs are the direct result of the doctor's lack of knowledge or skill (Doctor's Educational Needs; DENs). The PUNs and DENs method is focused around a logbook of patient contacts.

Having identified and written down the PUNs, the doctor considers *why* the patient's needs went unmet, annotates the deficiencies identified in him, or herself, and writes down an action plan to remedy the situation. Logbooks, instruction and examples can be obtained directly from Dr Richard Eve (eve97@msn.com) for a small charge. Alternatively, there are several good published summaries of the method available.[4]

Problem case analysis

Problem case analysis is very much an extension of PUNs and DENs. The registrar brings along the records of patients that are interesting or causing difficulties and the trainer and registrar discuss the learning needs that arose and how to deal with them. Such discussions are frequently wide-ranging and might end up covering areas of need far distant from the original perceived problem.

Random case analysis

The registrar brings to a tutorial the notes of a complete surgery. Early on in training this enables the trainer to keep track of how the registrar is coping. Later, it is useful to ensure that an adequate case mix is being seen. Each patient is a potential learning experience, and through Socratic dialogue[5] with the trainer, hitherto undiscovered learning needs can be revealed and the motivation to satisfy those needs enhanced.

Significant event analysis

Significant event analysis (SEA)[6] is a quick way of getting to those learning needs in the 'hidden' box of Johari's window. Crudely speaking it is a way of learning from our mistakes. The registrar, trainer or another member of the practice team raises an event as significant, such as a missed diagnosis, death of a patient or a practice complaint. All the parties involved discuss why the event is considered significant and determine the facts of the case. The important issues raised by the event are teased out. Those things that went well are highlighted together with those that went badly. Feasible areas for improvement are identified and an action plan drawn up. The SEA can then be written up and filed in the learning log or PDP. The key features of success of SEA are that:

- it should be a positive experience for all involved
- it should result in some improvement in patient care
- it is about improvement and development – not blame.

Feedback from patients, staff and colleagues

During the registrar year you will be working as part of a team. As such you will be working closely with your trainer, practice nurses, receptionists and the rest of the primary healthcare team. Each member of the team will have the opportunity to observe you in action and these observations will be fed back to you from time to time by your trainer.

A simple means of rapidly collecting information on your performance is the Follow-Up Slip System (FUSS). FUSS cards, downloadable from the London Deanery website (www. londondeanery.ac.uk), are lodged in the notes of, say 100, consecutive patients and pulled out and completed by the next doctor seeing the patient. That doctor comments on the diagnosis, management and patient's impression of the previous consultation. Once 100 completed cards have been returned they can be analysed for meaningful and instructive trends: for instance, there might be recurring mistakes in dermatological diagnosis. Issues arising from the analysis can then be discussed with the trainer and the appropriate remedial action taken.

Feedback can be given, and accepted, well or badly. Ideally, your trainer will give positive feedback where it is due and strive to achieve mutual agreement with you when offering constructive criticism. When things aren't going so well, it is helpful for the trainer to know if there are any external factors, e.g. domestic problems, that might be affecting your performance at work.

Patients are also a valuable source of feedback and you might canvass their views by utilising a patient satisfaction questionnaire. Formal instruments such as the Howie enablement questionnaire[7] might be useful in this respect.

Appraisals

An appraisal is a formative assessment process culminating in an interview performed by the trainer, course organiser or another. It gives the registrar an opportunity for feedback on the educational experience, as well as providing a forum to review what has been accomplished and plan for future learning.

Appraisals are about 'praise' and development and should not be used as a time for the appraiser, or appraisee, to dump all that negative stuff that has been building up for months.

An appraisal should end with a mutually-agreed statement of where future energies should be directed and an action plan. Objectives should be SMART: specific, measurable, attainable, resourced and time-bound. Many formal structures have been drawn up for such a statement and it may be that your training scheme has developed its own. One good generic example is the Mutually Agreed Reporting System (MARS) formally developed in South West Thames and available from the London Deanery website. Further discussion about appraisal in the context of continuing professional development (CPD) is to be found in Chapter 5.

Consultation analysis

Reviewing oneself on video tape can be a sobering but illuminating experience and there are many ways of enhancing this process including consultation mapping, consultation modelling and measurement against predetermined assessment instruments. With the shift in emphasis to video as an end-point assessment, it is easy to forget what a wonderful instructional tool video can be. Mutual exploration of the issues generated by a single videoed consultation remains one of the most powerful formative tools available in GP training. You can be sure that you and your trainer will be watching a lot of them.

Joint surgeries

Joint surgeries are fruitful when it comes to identifying learning needs but having your trainer sitting in the corner is a daunting prospect and can affect both the process and the outcome of the consultation. Patients also find it hard to ignore the fact that a more experienced and a more familiar doctor is in the room and may begin to address their enquiries in that direction.

Audit

Audit compares our performance against a set of criteria and standards. Audit is a powerful tool for learning in that it is about what we *actually* do, not what we say we do. The summative assessment process includes a requirement for a written submission of practical work, which is usually presented as a completed audit cycle. Conducting small-scale focused audits on a regular basis is a very good habit to get into and a sure-fire way of identifying our failings and improving the quality of care that we deliver.

Multiple choice questions (MCQs)

Mechanically marked multiple choice papers are probably the best method of testing knowledge. Both SA and the MRCGP examination include MCQ papers. Increasingly, however, such structured objective assessments are moving away from simple true–false statements to more complex question formats such as extended matching questions and single and multiple best answer questions. These novel formats are more capable of testing the understanding and application of knowledge rather than just factual acquisition itself.

Past MRCGP examination papers are obtainable from the sales office of the RCGP along with a CD-ROM phased evaluation programme (PEP) which offers objective assessment in a number of GP-relevant areas. The PEP also provides a facility whereby you can compare your own performance against previous attempts by registrars elsewhere in the country.

Modified essay questions

The modified essay question (MEQ) is an invention of the RCGP that has been used widely in other medical examinations. An MEQ consists of a scenario or situation in general practice followed by a short but searching question stem. For example:

> Daisy Boyd, aged 68 years, arrives late for her routine appointment smelling of urine. How would you manage this situation?

Each question is capable of testing a wide range of issues and the ability to think laterally, itself a core skill of general practice. For instance, the above question might raise issues as diverse as the management of incontinence through the management of time to the management of the doctor's own feelings. MEQs are a useful supplement to the kaleidoscopic parade of real patients and attendant problems that pass through our doors every day.

OSCEs and simulated surgeries

Objective structured clinical examinations (OSCEs) are being used increasingly as end-point assessments at medical school. The student, or in this case, GP registrar, is consulted by a carefully rehearsed simulated patient and a marking schedule prepared in advance for scoring the way the consultation is handled. OSCE stations are difficult to set up and maintain reliably but can provide a useful formative experience and are fun, particularly if there are two registrars in the practice. Examples of patient-orientated OSCE stations are to be found on the London Deanery website.

Personality profiles and self-perception tools

The attributes of a good GP are many and varied and include a host of elements that are not directly linked to the clinical care of patients but have a huge impact on how a particular individual works within the practice setting. Validated self-assessment questionnaires are extremely useful in beginning to understand more about oneself and can be used to look at such diverse attributes as team role,[8] learning styles[9] and personality type.[10] It is a good idea to complete these questionnaires at the same time as your trainer and the results may help the two of you to understand your own relationship better.

Logbooks, diaries and personal development plans

With all the assessments discussed it is a good idea to write down the results and action points arising. Apart from anything else, you'll forget what it was that was so important to learn last week when confronted by this week's agenda! A learning log or plan will help you to keep on track and will provide you with a basis for discussion when you undergo your regular appraisals during your registrar year.

Apart from these, a personal development plan (PDP) is a good habit to get into, as very soon, all GPs will be expected to have one. A detailed discussion of PDPs is to be found in Chapter 5 of this book. If you need further help, your trainer should have one and be able to advise you. Alternatively consult the London Deanery website (www.londondeanery.ac.uk) for a selection of model PDPs.

References

1   Middleton P and Field S (2001) *The GP Trainer's Handbook*. Radcliffe Medical Press, Oxford.

2   RCGP (1989) *Rating Scales for Vocational Training in General Practice*. Occasional Paper No. 40. Royal College of General Practitioners, London.

3   Eve R (2003) *PUNs & DENs*. Radcliffe Medical Press, Oxford.

4   Rughani A (2000) *PUNS & DENS*. In: *The GP's Guide to Personal Development Plans*. Radcliffe Medical Press, Oxford, pp. 91–9.

5   Neighbour R (1995) *The Inner Apprentice*. Kluwer Academic, London.

6   Pringle M, Bradley C, Carmichael C, Wallis H and Moore A (1995) *Significant Event Auditing*. Occasional Paper No. 75. Royal College of General Practitioners, London.

7   Howie JG, Heaney DJ and Maxwell M (1997) *Measuring Quality in General Practice: pilot study of a needs, process and outcome measure*. Occasional Paper. Royal College of General Practitioners, London.

8   Belbin RM (1981) *Management Teams: why they succeed or fail*. Heinemann Professional Publishing, Oxford.

9   Honey P and Mumford A (1992) *The Manual of Learning Styles*. Peter Honey, Maidenhead.

10 Myers Briggs I (1998) *Introduction to Type*. Oxford Psychologists Press, Oxford.

3

Summative assessment and the MRCGP examination

Two possible end-point assessments exist for general practice (GP) training. Summative assessment (SA) is required by law and is a test of fitness for independent practice; as such its standards are low but the stakes are high! Failing SA may necessitate remedial training as you cannot obtain your Certificate of Satisfactory Completion, and therefore set out on your own, without it.

The membership examination of the Royal College of General Practitioners (MRCGP) by contrast is a high standards examination, but at the time of writing, entirely voluntary. It is likely that at some point in the not too distant future these two end-point assessments will be merged together.

Summative assessment

What is summative assessment?

SA was introduced as a legal requirement of vocational training in 1997. It aims to provide objective evidence that registrars completing training have achieved a minimum level of competence, so enabling practice as independent general practitioners in the

NHS. As it is a test of minimum competence, SA should present no difficulty to the vast majority of GP registrars.

What does it involve?

SA has four elements and you must pass all four. These are:

*   a multiple choice question paper (MCQ)
*   an assessment of consulting skills
*   a written submission of practical work
*   a structured trainer's report.

Within the four components is a degree of choice. For instance, you might decide to sit a simulated surgery examination rather than submit video evidence of your consulting skills. Once all four components have been successfully completed, your trainer will sign a VTR1 form. This, together with the VTR2 forms from your hospital jobs, should be sent to the Deanery Summative Assessment administrator where they will be checked, endorsed and forwarded to the Joint Committee of Postgraduate Training for General Practice (JCPTGP), who in turn will issue a Statement of Satisfactory Completion. Certification is soon to come within the remit of the Postgraduate Medical Education and Training Board (PMETB).

How do I start?

A full and detailed description of the requirements and process of SA will be sent to you at the beginning of your registrar year together with your National Summative Assessment Number. Make a note of this. Take some time to read through the national guidance with your trainer and decide which of the various methods of assessment you wish to opt for. Having done this, complete your SA application form and return it to your deanery SA administrator (*see* Planning your summative assessment year, p. 22).

The MCQ

This machine-marked examination is set at the level of medical school finals, and is held four times each year. There are around 300 items for which you are allowed three hours. There is no negative marking. The pass rate is currently around 94% but should you fail, you may rc-sit the examination at the next available opportunity. As an alternative you may wish to sit the MCQ paper of the MRCGP examination. A pass automatically exempts you from the summative assessment MCQ. Details can be obtained from the examination office of the Royal College of General Practitioners (RCGP).

The written submission of practical work

The written submission is commonly referred to as 'the audit' because this is the assessment chosen by the majority of registrars and the favoured method in most deaneries. A completed audit cycle, including the implementation of change and a second collection of data, is required. The 'eight criteria audit' comes highly recommended, not only on educational grounds but because it presents an opportunity to have a real impact on your training practice. The golden rule here is 'keep it simple'. Avoid being over-ambitious. A small, well-focused and relevant audit will take less time to prepare and is more likely to bring about change. Avoid group audits with other registrars and follow-on audits from work already in progress within the practice.

As an alternative strategy, you may submit a variety of written projects under the National Project Marking Schedule (NPMS). Under the NPMS, many alternative project formats are permitted, from case reports to controlled trials. It has been proposed that the NPMS will become the written assessment of choice in the English deaneries in the near future. Application details are to be found in the National Summative Assessment Guide and on the website of the National Office for Summative Assessment (NOSA).

The assessment of consulting skills

There are currently three approved assessments of consulting skills:

- submit a video for SA purposes only
- submit a video for the consulting skills module of the MRCGP examination
- apply to have your skills tested by a simulated patient surgery.

The video required for SA should be recorded on VHS 'standard play' and contain two hours of (a minimum of eight) consultations. The tape should demonstrate your performance at a varied level of challenge. An accompanying logbook provides a chance to explain the circumstances of the consultation and what you were doing. You are not asked to submit a master-piece, but the consultation must be free from major errors that might put a patient at risk or collections of minor errors that might cause inconvenience or embarrassment.

A more challenging and potentially more satisfying video assessment is the consulting skills module of the MRCGP examination. Again the bare bones of an effective consultation are covered, but you will also be required to demonstrate a patient-centred consulting style. Like the MCQ, a pass in the MRCGP video module gains exemption from SA. Should you not be successful, your videotape will be automatically 'fast-tracked' through local SA procedures. Over 90% of candidates who fail the MRCGP video will go on to pass SA.

Details of the simulated patient surgeries held in the Yorkshire and mid-Trent deaneries are to be found in the National Summative Assessment Guide and on the website of NOSA.

The trainer's report

The final piece in the SA jigsaw, the trainer's report, is a comprehensive summary of your clinical and organisational skills, your ability to diagnose and manage patients, as well as an assessment of your professional values and personal and professional growth. Trainers should point out identified weaknesses during your training period, allowing time and plenty of support to work on those areas that you might find more difficult. If you're not sure how things are going – ask.

When do I get my results?

Results will be sent out by your deanery summative assessment administrator by letter, and will not generally be given over the telephone. You can expect to receive them as indicated below:

- MCQ – at least three weeks after the examination
- Audit – five weeks after receipt by the deanery
- Video – eight weeks after receipt by the deanery.

How do I appeal?

If you are unhappy with the way your SA submissions were processed, there is an appeals procedure, a copy of which can be obtained from your deanery summative assessment administrator. If you think that you have under-performed for some other reason, e.g. illness, transport delays, you can lodge an appeal with the deanery but only before the results have been made available.

What if I fail?

The vast majority of registrars pass SA, but in the unlikely event of failure, additional training time within the deanery, usually up to a maximum of six months, can be made available. If you are having problems along the way, discuss them as early as possible with your trainer and course organiser. They are there to help – use them!

Planning your summative assessment year

Month 1   Read the SA guidance that has been sent to you thoroughly. Study the National Trainer's Report so that you know what will be expected of you by the end of the year.

Month 2   Check when and where the next MCQ is being held. Taking the MCQ during your first three months is not recommended.

Month 3   Complete and return the SA application form, which includes an indication of when you will be sitting your MCQ. Start thinking about suitable subjects for your written submission. If opting for the completed audit cycle, remember that you will need to collect two rounds of data and that the finished audit will need to be in by the end of Month 9. It's best to start early. This also applies to videoing your consultations!

Month 5   You should be well on the way to completing your video and audit. If confident, attempt the MCQ this month.

Month 6   The video and audit should be submitted between now and Month 9. Don't leave it too late as you may have trouble if you don't pass first time. If sitting the MRCGP examination, apply by the end of this month.

Month 8   The deadline for submitting the single route MRCGP/SA video is this month. Simulated surgeries are held between Month 8 and 10.

Month 9   The deadline for the COGPED video and audit is the end of this month.

Month 11   Your trainer should submit the trainer's report this month together with a signed VTR1.

Month 12   JCPTGP issues a Statement of Satisfactory Completion.

The membership examination of the Royal College of General Practitioners

The examination for membership (MRCGP) is a credit accumulation examination. There are four modules which may be taken, and hopefully passed, in any order, at any time within three years of your initial application. The examination changes with alarming regularity so it will be worth your while obtaining the current regulations from the RCGP. Information about the examination is also available on the RCGP website www.rcgp.org.uk. A comprehensive syllabus outlining the scope of the MRCGP examination will soon be available.

The four modules of the MRCGP examination are:

- a written paper
- a multiple choice paper
- an assessment of consulting skills
- an oral examination.

In addition to the above, you must also provide evidence of proficiency in basic cardiopulmonary resuscitation and child health surveillance.

The written paper

Both the written paper and the MCQ are available twice a year. The written paper's main aim according to the college regulations is 'to examine your ability to integrate and apply theoretical knowledge and professional values within the setting of primary healthcare in the United Kingdom'. Although a content review of the examination is underway at present, the main themes of the written paper are currently:

- consultation-based problem solving, informed decision making and clinical management

- consultation and communication skills
- evidence-based practice in the treatment and prevention of disease
- critical appraisal
- challenges and dilemmas in practice
- values sensitivity and empathy
- responsibilities to partners, other health professionals and society.

Questions come in a variety of formats ranging from scenario-based modified essay questions to the analysis of extracts of published papers. Examples of all types of questions are published in the examination regulations, and the RCGP website displays past written paper questions alongside examiners' comments about how each question might best have been answered.

The multiple choice paper

The multiple choice or machine-marked module is designed to test your knowledge of core and emerging general practice, and more importantly, the deeper understanding and application of that knowledge. The content areas are:

- medicine
- administration and management
- research epidemiology and statistics.

Again, full details are to be found in the examination regulations.

Much more than multiple choice, this machine-marked paper is host to an array of novel question formats. The paper no longer includes the true–false statements that we are all familiar with, but tests understanding and application much more effectively with extended matching questions, single and multiple best answer questions, and questions involving summary and algorithm completion. Tables and data are presented within the paper, along with photographs and electrocardiograms.

Consulting skills

There are two distinct assessments of consulting skills in the examination. The default assessment is a video submission, but a simulated surgery is available for candidates who have 'insuperable difficulty in submitting a video tape for assessment'. The video assessment is based on the concept of competency. A list of consulting competencies have been identified and from these distilled a marking schedule of performance criteria. You are asked to demonstrate that you can exhibit the various competencies within seven selected recorded consultations. The requirements are laid out in fine detail in the RCGP *Video Assessment of Consulting Skills – Workbook and Instructions*. Read them!

Oral examination

The oral examination assesses your decision making and the professional values underpinning those decisions. Questions are posed in two separate 20-minute orals by two pairs of examiners. To ensure a spread of question subjects, examiners are asked to assess communication, professional values and personal and professional growth across four contexts:

- care of patients
- working with colleagues
- the social role of general practice
- the doctor's personal responsibilities.

This is one part of the examination where strategic preparation will pay off. Find a friendly examiner and practice answering some questions – picking your way through ethical dilemmas under pressure may not come naturally!

How do I apply?

Application forms and full details are available from the Examination Department of the RCGP. You can apply for all modules together or singly over the three-year permitted period.

Please note that before taking up College membership you must have received your Certificate of Satisfactory Completion from the JCPTGP, and in order to attain this, you must have satisfied the requirements of SA.

Useful addresses

National Office of Summative Assessment
King Alfred's College
Winchester
Hants SO22 4NR

Tel: 01962 827389
www.nosa.org.uk

JCPTGP and RCGP
14 Princes Gate
London SW7 1PU

Tel: 020 7581 3232
www.rcgp.org.uk
www.jcptgp.org.uk

4

Teaching and learning in general practice

When we visit training practices for the purposes of trainer reaccredidation, the registrars we interview are asked about the teaching they receive. At the same visit, trainers are quizzed about the education and training they provide. Surprisingly, there is often a discrepancy in these accounts and it appears that although there may be a wealth of learning opportunities offered to registrars, not all of it is registered, or recalled, by the learners as education that 'counts'. There are some perfectly understandable reasons for this which will briefly be explored in this chapter, as we highlight some key concepts of adult learning theory and how these theoretical models apply to the training year. We hope that this chapter will give you some insight into the educational and developmental processes at work during your training, and by doing so, help you gain the most from your experience.

Adult learning

One of the many advantages that children have over adults is the ability to remember what they are taught. Children are also easily captivated and motivated, and to a certain extent, manipulated in learning situations. Adults, by contrast, struggle to embrace new concepts and to assimilate new knowledge, a

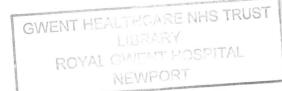

problem made more acute in medicine where we have to recall and apply what we know in unpredictable, and unforeseen, high stakes situations. Our predicament is that of the cartoonist Gary Larson's rather mangy and worried looking hound. High on a tightrope above a torrential Niagara Falls, 'Rex', writes Larson, 'was an old dog, and it was a new trick'.

Throughout the past century, various educators in Europe and America examined the way in which adults tended to function most effectively in the learning situation. Common themes emerged which were pulled together in the 1970s by Malcolm Knowles in his classic book *The Adult Learner: a neglected species*.[1] Knowles is best known for coining the term *androgogy*, to distinguish the learning processes that adults engage in, as distinct to *pedagogy* – the pouring of knowledge into the receptive and empty vessels of children's minds or 'jugs to mugs'. Adult learning, summarises Knowles, is most effective when it is:

- self-directed
- experiential
- needs-based
- problem-centred.

Self-directed learning

As an individual grows and matures, his or her self-concept moves from one of total dependency to increasing self-directedness. A person psychologically becomes an adult when they achieve self-direction. There is a deep-seated need for adults to be self-directed, and if they are not allowed to be so, tension, resentment and resistance will result. In other words, as an adult, you're in charge, and you will want to remain in charge, of your own learning.

Self-direction is not a concept that comes easily to some, and most of us, faced with new situations will want to be told what to do rather than have to find out for ourselves. This tension was described by an American psychologist, William Perry, who examined the emotional relationship to learning of a cohort of students at Harvard University.[2] He found a progression from 'dualism' to 'relativism', a gradual shaking off over time, of a dependence on the teacher, leading to a mature, adult position of self-reliance with its attendant acceptance of the complex and confusing nature of the world. Figure 4.1 is taken from Perry's work and describes this progression as applied to general practice (GP) training. Where are you on this journey? Does your trainer know best – or is he as confused as you are?

Experiential learning

Experience provides the principal adult resource for learning. Adults have a broad base of experience and it is into this bedrock that they sink, or 'connect' new ideas. Furthermore, adults define themselves by their experience, that is to say, what we have done, or what we do, is extremely important to our self-belief. If this experience is ignored or undervalued, an adult will feel neglected as a person.

Experiential learning is also an iterative process, situations can be revisited again and again and something new can be gained each time. As TS Eliot succinctly describes:[3]

> We shall not cease from exploration
> And the end of all our exploring
> Will be to arrive where we started
> And know the place for the first time.

In other words, as a GP registrar you bring a huge quantity of prior and highly relevant experience to your training year. Adult learning connects up those experiences with new ones and in doing so provides you with a fresh outlook on old situations.

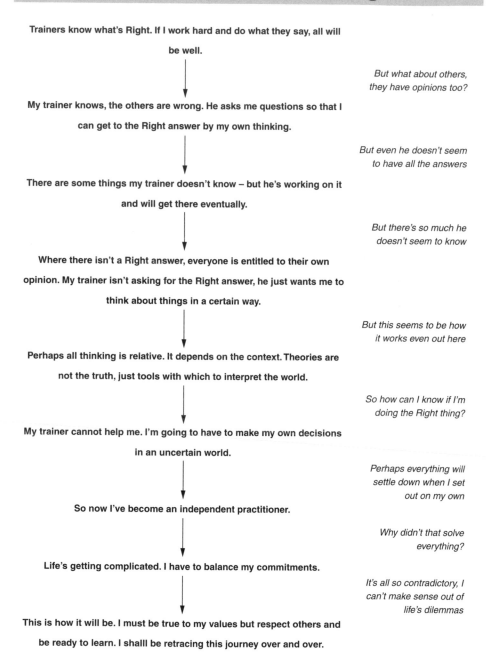

Trainers know what's Right. If I work hard and do what they say, all will be well.

But what about others, they have opinions too?

My trainer knows, the others are wrong. He asks me questions so that I can get to the Right answer by my own thinking.

But even he doesn't seem to have all the answers

There are some things my trainer doesn't know – but he's working on it and will get there eventually.

But there's so much he doesn't seem to know

Where there isn't a Right answer, everyone is entitled to their own opinion. My trainer isn't asking for the Right answer, he just wants me to think about things in a certain way.

But this seems to be how it works even out here

Perhaps all thinking is relative. It depends on the context. Theories are not the truth, just tools with which to interpret the world.

So how can I know if I'm doing the Right thing?

My trainer cannot help me. I'm going to have to make my own decisions in an uncertain world.

Perhaps everything will settle down when I set out on my own

So now I've become an independent practitioner.

Why didn't that solve everything?

Life's getting complicated. I have to balance my commitments.

It's all so contradictory, I can't make sense out of life's dilemmas

This is how it will be. I must be true to my values but respect others and be ready to learn. I shall be retracing this journey over and over.

Figure 4.1: Emotional relationships to learning in the GP registrar year. (From Perry W (1970) Forms of intellectual and ethical development in the college years.[2])

Needs-based learning

An adult's readiness to learn is the product of the developmental tasks required for the performance of his or her evolving social roles. We learn best when the circumstances we find ourselves in make it necessary for us to do so. In GP training, there is a readiness to learn about different issues at different stages and a typical curriculum of learning needs, or learning 'trajectory' develops throughout the training period. On the day-to-day level, there is also a hunger for new knowledge and skills driven by the discomfort that is generated by situations where we find ourselves struggling, or simply just don't know the answer. Sensitising yourself to these moments of discomfort, or need, is vital to your continuing professional development, and your trainer will ensure – in the nicest possible way of course – that these moments are brought to your attention. 'Confusion' as the nuclear physicist Edmund Teller once said 'is not a bad thing – it's the first step towards understanding'.

Problem-centred learning

An adult comes into an educational activity largely because of some perceived inadequacy in coping with current life problems. We want to apply tomorrow what we learn today. The appropriate units for adult teaching and learning are therefore *not* subjects, but situations. If you were expecting a set tutorial every week on all the major chronic diseases, this news may be disappointing, but ultimately you will find problem-centred teaching and learning much more rewarding.

Take diabetes for example. You are visited by a patient with poorly controlled type I disease. You stall for time and arrange some blood tests but they are coming back tomorrow and you need to know how to go about changing their insulin regime. A conversation takes place between you and your trainer in the corridor, followed by a telephone discussion with the diabetic liaison nurse at the hospital and you read the relevant section of the *BNF* over coffee. You formulate a plan for your patient. Learning has taken place because you needed to know, you needed to know at that moment, and you are able to apply that knowledge immediately.

However, one doesn't have to wait passively for readiness to happen. It can be stimulated and another of your trainer's tasks will be to supply that stimulation, providing a graded exposure to the increasingly complex and wide-ranging discipline of general practice.

The learning cycle

So how does it work in practice, this self-directed, experiential, needs-based, problem-centred learning? And what about all that recommended reading?

David Kolb[4] described a process of experiential learning which is depicted graphically in Figure 4.2. In this *learning cycle* the adult learner has an experience, comes away and reflects on that experience, tries to make sense of what happened on the basis of theoretical considerations available to them, and connects up what happened with what they already know. Then, equipped for the future, the adult learner prepares for the next experience. And so it goes.

Take a typical consultation in a perfectly ordinary surgery. Mrs Smith asks you whether you think Jade should be referred for grommets. You bluster your way through the consultation and afterwards, on reflection, decide that your discussion of the options was probably inadequate for her needs. You go to the library and conduct a search of the available evidence. As a result you produce a short leaflet for the practice which you intend to use in a subsequent consultation. Experience has led

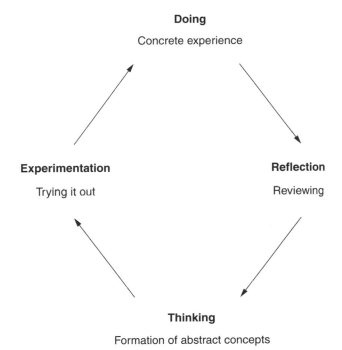

Figure 4.2: The Kolb learning cycle.

to reflection, to theoretical exploration, and to preparation for the next experience. In other words, you have now completed one turn around the learning cycle. However, the next time the grommet question arises, despite your leaflet, the consultation takes a different turn and revolves around the parent's insistence on the use of homeopathy to treat her child's glue ear. Reflective discussion with your trainer this time takes you down the road of ethics and health beliefs. Another learning cycle begins.

Donald Schön developed a similar model to the Kolb cycle that he identified in self-educating professionals.[5] This he termed *reflective practice*, a process engaged in by the *reflective practitioner*. In Schön's *reflection in action:*

- the practitioner spontaneously initiates a routine action that produces an unexpected outcome – Surprise!

- the surprise is noticed as an error, an anomaly, an opportunity
- reflection triggered
- understanding of situation restructured
- new strategy invented
- on-the-spot experimentation which leads to a satisfactory outcome *or*
- … another surprise.

Another example: A hesitant Debbie comes to see you about her crying baby. After a slightly dysfunctional start to the consultation and unsure as to what to say, you fall silent. Tearfully she opens up and begins to tell you about the problems the baby is causing with her marriage. Gosh – not jumping in and involving the health visitor immediately seems to have reaped rewards. You reflect on what has happened and realise that had you pursued your normal course of offering advice, this outpouring may never have happened. Perhaps you are cutting patients off too quickly in your anxiety to solve their problems. You decide to use silence more often in your consultations and see where it gets you.

General practice is full of surprises. Make the most of them.

Learning styles

Not everyone likes to learn in the same way, and we each have a preference for a particular phase of the learning cycle. Some of us prefer to learn by getting stuck in, others by quietly reflecting on what has happened. It may be that you prefer to read around a subject in a book, whilst a colleague might only be interested in a topic if it is of immediate and practical relevance. It is important to know your preferred learning style and to be aware of those styles that *don't* come so naturally – to be an effective learner you need to cultivate them all.

Several tools exist for determining your own preferred learning style[6] and your trainer or course organiser should be able to point you in the direction of a learning styles questionnaire.

Expectations of teaching

So what can you expect of the teaching you receive and the learning you undertake in general practice?

You can look forward to a seemingly chaotic programme of patient-orientated, problem-based learning with teaching episodes focused on the burning issues of that day. These may occur at any time of day, or night. Sure, there will be set-piece tutorials, but it is quite likely that you will be the one giving them.

You will be given the opportunity to try out new knowledge and skills in a supportive environment and will be provided with the time and space to reflect on your experiences.

When appropriate, your trainer will provide you with theoretical frameworks by which to organise your thoughts, or at least you will be pointed in the direction of the right book.

Learning opportunities will present themselves in a myriad of different forms and most will not involve your trainer at all. All members of the practice and primary healthcare team will be involved in your learning. Be alert to every opportunity.

Throughout all this, your trainer will be on hand to ensure that you are safe, protected and supplied with the experiences you need, at the time that you need them.

And over time, you will be taken on an enabling journey of guided self-discovery, which, we hope, will result in your development as a motivated, mature and insightful adult learner.

References

1   Knowles M (1973) *The Adult Learner: a neglected species.* Gulf Publishing Company, Houston.

2   Perry W (1970) *Forms of Intellectual and Ethical Development in the College Years: a scheme.* Jossey-Bass, San Francisco.

3   Eliot TS (1963) *Four quartets.* In: *Collected Poems 1909–1962.* Faber, London.

4   Kolb DA (1984) *Experiential Learning: experience as a source of learning and development.* Prentice Hall, Englewood Cliffs, Chicago.

5   Schön D (1983) *The Reflective Practitioner.* Maurice Temple Smith, London.

6   Honey P and Mumford A (1992) *The Manual of Learning Styles.* Peter Honey, Maidenhead.

5

Continuing professional development

Continuing professional development (CPD) is an important aspect of the life of any general practitioner (GP). It represents a continuous and reflective process, maximising learning from the many sources and opportunities, which emerge in the working life of a GP.

In working through this study guide it is hoped that the reader will have engaged in a developmental journey, which has moved through three phases of learning namely:

- assessment of personal developmental needs
- designing a tailored learning programme
- reviewing of learning and the impact on the practice.

These phases will form the key stages of a personal development plan (PDP), which is essentially a practical and time-related action plan outlining the development of the individual. It is generally considered that the PDP will relate to one year's activity.

Before considering the practical elements involved in developing a PDP it is important to consider three important elements which will affect the development process:

- reflective learning
- mentorship
- GP appraisal.

Reflective learning

As discussed in Chapter 4, the most potent motivation to learn comes from the need to know. When adults experience uncertainty in their work this acts as a potent stimulus to learn. Experience alone does not, however, guarantee learning and it is necessary for learners to reflect on what they do, what they become aware of and what they feel before they can define their learning needs.[1]

Most learning in general practice is self-directed. Every day GPs will have experiences from which they could learn. Therefore the next skill necessary is to *prioritise* learning needs. The prioritisation process may be affected by many factors including the needs of the practice, as well as the primary care trust (PCT) and national priorities.

Mentoring

The term 'mentor' is one of those words used ubiquitously in general practice and means different things to different people. As scholars of the classics will remember, 'Mentor', in Greek mythology, was charged with the responsibility of looking after and bringing up the son of Ulysses as he went to fight in the Trojan Wars. Thus the role of a mentor may be considered to be paternalistic and supervisory for some, whereas to others a mentor may fulfil a more psychotherapeutic function. In educational terms a mentor can be considered an individual who facilitates the process of learning and provides support and counselling.[2]

So why is all this relevant? At some point in the planning or review process for a PDP it will be beneficial to get the support and guidance of someone with skills in observing and giving useful feedback on your activities. For most GP registrars this function may be fulfilled by his or her trainer. For others finding someone whose judgement you trust and who is appropriately skilled is the key. Remember that the skills needed include:

- confidential feedback
- support
- challenge
- recommendations for alternative ways of doing things.

Appraisal

It is worth mentioning at this stage that all GPs working in the NHS are to be appraised annually by GP appraisers appointed by their PCTs. The appraisal process will be formative and, after the appraisal has been completed, will lead to recommendations which can contribute to the subsequent year's PDP process. The system of annual appraisal for GPs will be linked to their five-yearly revalidation, or re-licensing.

Personal development plans made easy

Rughani[4] suggests answering the following questions when planning to write a PDP.

- What is the general area in which I need to learn?
- How have I established the need?
- What is the aim of my learning?
- What are the specific objectives that I wish to achieve?
- How do I intend to achieve these objectives?
- How will I evaluate my development plan?
- How will I demonstrate that I have undertaken this plan?

Ewan Armstrong[3] on behalf of the South Thames Deanery developed a practical guide for writing a PDP upon which this next section is largely based.

As identified earlier there are essentially three steps involved in an effective PDP process.

Step 1: Identifying your developmental needs.
Step 2: Designing a tailored learning programme.
Step 3: Reviewing the impact of learning on practice.

Step 1: Identifying your developmental needs

What is a developmental need?

Developmental needs may be *knowledge*-based, *skill*-based or *attitudinal*. The needs are identified as a discrepancy between where the doctor is and where he or she would like to be in order to deliver quality healthcare.

The identification of developmental or learning needs has already been covered in Chapter 2 of this guide. The following list is just a reminder of some triggers, which can help to identify developmental needs:

- self-awareness/confidence rating scales
- feedback from colleagues and patients
- feedback from appraisal
- significant event analysis (SEA)
- video-tapes of consultations
- analysis of patient contacts
  - contemporaneously, e.g. PUNs and DENs
  - retrospectively, e.g. SEA
- prescribing and practice activity (PACT) data
- objective tests, e.g. MCQs, evaluation programmes on CD
- educational meetings – identify issues raised during or after the meeting that suggest further educational needs
- replies to referral letters
- audit
- research.

Some practical considerations

- It is a good idea to collect information from a range of different sources to help identify needs over a period of say one or two months.
- Theme the information collected into needs in the areas of knowledge, skills or attitudes.
- Enlist the help of a colleague to help prioritise needs identified.

Turning needs into learning outcomes

Having prioritised the development needs, a particular challenge is converting them into learning outcomes. These are specific statements that will form the goals of the PDP.

The acronym **SMART** is a useful way of constructing learning outcomes. Learning outcomes should be:

Specific	Is the stated outcome as specific as possible?
Measurable	How would you check (by measurement, observation, feedback) whether the outcome had been achieved?
Achievable	Check resources (expertise, time, etc.) are available.
Realistic	Don't bite off more than you can chew!
Time-bounded	Set dates for completion of the outcome, e.g. 'by the end of a course of study ...'

Stage 2: Designing your learning programme

Having identified learning outcomes it is important to choose methods for achieving them which take into account your preferred learning style (*see* Chapter 4), personal circumstances, availability of resources and time.

Learning outcomes can be addressed using a variety of methods. Each has strengths and weaknesses and a selection of them are listed below. There is no right or wrong way to learn but two points are worth repeating. Firstly, learning is more effective when it is interactive and therefore doctors should resist the temptation to learn everything from a book or by sitting passively through a lecture. Secondly, learning is most often applied when it is relevant to the circumstances of a doctor's work. Therefore practice-based learning has much to recommend it.[1]

Learning methods

These include:

- reading: medical/non-medical
- the internet: good for quality, reliability and accessibility of information available
- lectures
- workshops
- courses
- multidisciplinary learning
- practice-based learning (e.g. SEA, audit, developing guidelines)
- distance learning
- skills training
- video analysis
- mentoring
- young principals' group
- Balint group.

Whilst it is important to take into account one's preferred learning style when addressing learning outcomes, it is also wise to choose different methods of learning as a variety of educational experience can be more stimulating. So a recommendation is to use at least two different methods of learning to address a specific learning outcome.

Step 3: Reviewing the impact of learning

As mentioned above when writing your PDP it is important to consider how the PDP will be reviewed or evaluated when setting out learning outcomes and developing the programme for learning. Take, for example, a section of a PDP designed to address a learning need around joint injections in general practice.

Aim

> To perform joint injections in general practice.

Specific learning outcomes

> By the end of the 2-month programme I will be able to:
>
> 1 Outline the main clinical indications and contraindications for injecting joints and trigger points.
> 2 Demonstrate adequate skills in performing injections.
> 3 Develop practice guidelines for performing injections.

Learning programme

Timing	Educational method	Learning outcome addressed	Evaluation
Week 1	Focused reading of relevant literature	1	Written report
Weeks 2–6	Sitting in rheumatology clinic with consultant	1, 2	Direct observation of injections, signed letter from consultant
Weeks 6–8	Multidisciplinary meeting	3	Draft guidelines established
Week 8	Practice guidelines at practice meeting	3	Guidelines agreed

Upon completion of a cycle of PDP activity it is important to reflect on whether the learning outcomes have been achieved by measuring your success against your original outcomes. It is worth reviewing whether the original outcomes were true reflections of learning needs and whether they were realistic. Evaluation of the methods of learning used, how effectively resources were used and whether there were any particular difficulties encountered along the way could also be part of the review. Getting feedback from a colleague can help with this process.

It is also important to review how the learning programme has changed your practice. Feedback from patients, staff, review of practice data and naturally personal reflections will form part of this. A short written report reviewing this stage of the PDP is a good way of ending this cycle of PDP activity.

The next stage is to celebrate your success in completing your PDP and start planning the next one!!

References

1   Gardiner P, Chana N and Jones R (2001) *An Insider's Guide to the MRCGP Oral Exam*. Radcliffe Medical Press, Oxford.

2   RCGP Working Group on Higher Education (1993) *Portfolio-based Learning in General Practice*. Occasional Paper No. 63. Royal College of General Practitioners, London.

3   Armstrong E (2000) *Personal Development Planning: a handbook for GPs*. South Thames Deanery, London.

4   Rughani A (2000) *The GP's Guide to Personal Development Plans*. Radcliffe Medical Press, Oxford.

Further reading

Lawrence M and Schofield T (1993) *Medical Audit in Primary Health Care*. Oxford General Practice Series No 25. Oxford University Press, Oxford.

Pendleton D and Hasler J (1997) *Professional Development in General Practice*. Oxford Medical Publications, Oxford.

Pringle M, Bradley C, Carmichael C, Wallis H and Moore A (1995) *Significant Event Auditing*. Occasional Paper No. 70. Royal College of General Practitioners, London.

Wakley G, Chambers R and Field S (2000) *Continuous Professional Development in Primary Care: making it happen*. Radcliffe Medical Press, Oxford.

While R and Attwood M (2000) *Professional Development: a guide for general practice*. Blackwell Science, Oxford.

6

The topic areas

This chapter, the core of this book, is essentially a curriculum for general practice. A curriculum is a plan of learning, that is, the *what*, the *how* and the *when*. The 22 topics have been derived from various key sources, including a syllabus drawn up by the examiners of the MRCGP, and comprehensively cover all aspects of general practice.

Each topic section is built on the same pattern, a brief introduction followed by three sections:

- what should be learned
- how to do it
- test yourself.

'What should be learned' states the intended learning outcomes or objectives. In places they are highly specific, in others quite general. This is deliberate. When you stumble across a phrase such as 'demonstrate an ability to diagnose and treat simple eye conditions', think about what these might be, ask your trainer and consult the appropriate GP-relevant literature. 'How to do it' lists some suggestions of ways to learn. The list is by no means exhaustive. Learning should be fun and, for adults, is best achieved under the conditions already extensively discussed in Chapter 4. Not all learning methods suit everyone but try to be open to as varied an educational diet as you can. 'Test yourself' is not an examination. These questions serve merely to stimulate thought, and perhaps discussion with your trainer or peers, around that particular topic area. If you want an assessment, Chapters 2 and 3 will tell you where to find one.

Topic 1 The nature of general practice

Traditionally a general practitioner gives personal, primary and continuing care to a small, relatively stable population. This compares with hospital-based care, which tends to be more episodic but is delivered to a much larger population. Increasingly in general practice, there has been a shift from the management of individuals to the management of small populations. The continuing care aspect of general practice requires the building of a special relationship with patients, which can have positive as well as negative elements. There is also a need to develop long-term relationships with colleagues, and managing these over a period of time requires special skills.

The way illness presents in primary care and the resources available may be very different to the hospital setting, therefore a complete understanding of the many issues currently facing GPs is vital for anyone contemplating a career in general practice. What really makes general practice challenging is dealing with uncertainty on a regular basis. As a result, there is the need to develop effective strategies for preventing harm to patients and learning from mistakes, thus effectively managing clinical risk. Finally, general practice imposes huge demands on our time and personal resources; achieving a balance between personal and working life is critically important.

What should be learned

At the end of training, the GP registrar will be able to:

- outline the varied professional roles undertaken by a general practitioner
- demonstrate the ability to manage both acute and continuing problems simultaneously
- demonstrate the ability to manage complex problems presenting in general practice

- carry out a focused assessment of a patient's condition, paying particular attention to the use of time and resources
- define personal strategies for managing uncertainty both within and outside of the consultation
- demonstrate an awareness of the limits of his/her professional competence
- demonstrate the ability to practise in such a way as to reduce the chance of harm occurring to patients
- demonstrate the ability to respond to criticisms or complaints appropriately and be able to learn from them
- demonstrate a flexible approach in dealing with patients according to patient need.

How to do it

- Discussion with your trainer and peers about the role of a GP.
- Small group discussion on the vocational training scheme (VTS) day-release course will enable greater understanding of the many issues currently facing GPs and enable sharing of the feelings generated when faced with uncertainty in the consultation. Traditionally in half-day release schemes, these discussions have taken place in smaller Balint-style groups.
- Direct observation of your trainer and other GPs within the practice to understand the GP style of consultation.
- Video consultation analysis with your trainer is an effective way of learning new strategies by analysing what you actually do.
- Reflection on personal experience whilst doing the job. Keeping a daily log of consultations and discussing interesting or challenging ones with your trainer.
- Review any complaints or criticisms with your trainer and identify any areas for improvement.

Reading

The selected reading shown here will give you a better understanding of general practice.

Fry J (1983) *The Future General Practitioner.* Royal College of General Practitioners, London.

Fry J (1999) *Common Diseases, their Nature, Incidence and Care (5e).* Librapharm/Petroc Press, Newbury.

Heath I (1995) *The Mystery of General Practice.* Nuffield Provincial Hospitals Trust, London.

Helman C (1990) *Culture, Health and Illness.* Butterworth-Heinemann, Oxford.

Lane K (1992) *The Longest Art.* Royal College of General Practitioners, London.

Pringle M (1998) *Core Values in Primary Care.* BMJ Books, London.

Qureshi B (1998) *Transcultural Medicine: dealing with patients from different cultures.* Librapharm/Petroc Press, Newbury.

Rakel R (2002) *Textbook of Family Practice (6e).* WB Saunders Co., Philadelphia.

Rosenthal J, Naish J and Lloyd M (1994) *The Trainee's Companion to General Practice.* Churchill Livingstone, Edinburgh.

Simon C, Everitt H, Birtwisle J and Stevenson B (2002) *The Oxford Handbook of General Practice.* Oxford University Press, Oxford.

Test yourself

What are the various roles undertaken by a GP? Which of these could be dealt with by another professional?

What could you realistically hope to achieve in a 10-minute consultation with a patient presenting with symptoms suggestive of chronic fatigue syndrome for the first time?

Outline some consultations that have left you feeling uncertain. Why has this happened? How did you cope?

What is the practice's procedure for dealing with complaints?

What have you learned from any criticisms or complaints made against you personally?

Topic 2 The consultation

After a few weeks in general practice it may dawn on you that the traditional medical model of history, diagnosis, investigation and treatment just doesn't work. Patients come with lists of problems, or they won't tell you what is really wrong, they've got funny ideas about their illness and sometimes days go by without a recognisable diagnosis being made. Some patients won't do what you tell them and some never come back. Others come back far too often. You need some other, more effective ways of handling patients in consultations. Fortunately, general practitioners have been looking at the consultation for decades, a wealth of literature exists on the subject, and a large proportion of your training year will be spent examining these frustrating and fascinating encounters.

What should be learned

At the end of training, the GP registrar will be able to:

- demonstrate good communication and consultation skills and show familiarity with the well-recognised consultation models
- respect the experience of patients, their ideas, concerns and expectations and also their dignity
- conduct patient-centred consultations involving and empowering the patient as a partner in care
- effectively develop ongoing relationships with patients whilst being aware of professional boundaries
- adapt the consultation process to the needs of different patients
- analyse the feelings of the patient and doctor in the consultation and have an insight into the psychological processes at play in the doctor–patient relationship

- understand the factors in consultations which are associated with better patient outcomes
- manage time and resources effectively within the consultation
- deal with patients effectively and safely using the telephone.

How to do it

- Observe your trainer and the other partners in the practice at work.
- Hold joint surgeries with your trainer.
- Discuss and analyse video recordings of your consultations with your trainer.
- Participate in small group discussions about consultations and the feelings generated by them.
- Engage in group analysis of recordings, e.g. at half-day release or on consultation courses. This is probably the best method.

Reading

Balint M (1957) *The Doctor, his Patient and the Illness*. Pitman Medical, London.

Bendix T (1982) *The Anxious Patient*. Churchill Livingstone, London.

Berne E (1966) *Games People Play*. Andre Deutsch, London.

Neighbour RH (1987) *The Inner Consultation*. MTP Press, Lancaster.

Pendleton D, Schofield T, Tate P *et al.* (1984) *The Consultation: an approach to learning and teaching*. Oxford University Press, Oxford.

Silverman J, Kurtz S and Draper J (1998) *Skills for Communicating with Patients*. Radcliffe Medical Press, Oxford.

Tate P (1997) *The Doctor's Communication Handbook*. Radcliffe Medical Press, Oxford.

Test yourself

Why do some consultations go wrong?

Are your patients satisfied with your consultations? How do/would you know?

Are you able to keep up a reasonable pace of consultation and are you able to achieve all that you would like to in your consultations. If not, why not?

Think of a patient that you find difficult. Are you able to understand your feelings and those of the patient?

What lessons can you learn from applying consultation models when watching your consultations?

What are your strengths and weaknesses in communication with patients?

Topic 3 Psychosocial disease in general practice

Psychosocial problems are extremely common in general practice. Approximately one third of consultations may have a psychosocial basis. Managing this large area of general practice requires effective interpersonal skills and an awareness of one's own attitudes in addition to having an adequate knowledge base. Whilst knowledge and skills can be learned, attitudinal change is much more difficult, so it is particularly important to try to understand the opinions and attitudes of other members of the primary and secondary care teams in order to develop your own perspective.

What should be learned

At the end of training, the GP registrar will be able to:

- interpret symptoms gathered from the patient in physical, psychological, social and cultural terms
- demonstrate an awareness of how psychodynamic factors, either individual or within the family can play a role in the development of mental disorder
- describe the natural history, clinical features and management of
  - depression, including assessment of suicidal risk
  - anxiety states
  - major mental illness including psychotic disorders such as schizophrenia
  - obsessional neurosis and other commoner psychiatric conditions
  - sleep disorders
  - learning difficulties and mental disability
  - eating disorders
- develop skills in the recognition and management of somatisation and personality disorders

- state the main provisions of the Mental Health Act
- describe the management of acute psychiatric emergencies
- outline the management of a psychosocial crisis
- describe the main drug dependency and substance abuse problems that may occur in practice and outline personal strategies for coping with these
- state the basic pharmacology of commonly used psychotropic drugs and the indication for their usage in specific circumstances
- describe the theoretical basis of the main psychological treatments used in general practice, their indications for use and their limitations
- demonstrate basic skills in supportive counselling and behavioural therapy
- describe the roles of other professionals concerned with mental health and state the indications for referral to them
- outline strategies for mental health promotion in different patient groups, e.g. adolescents, post-natal patients, elderly, refugees, asylum seekers.

How to do it

- Directly observe your trainer and other partners in the practice.
- Video analysis of psychological consultations with your trainer.
- Small group discussion on the day-release course of your VTS will allow an opportunity to explore personal attitudes to patients suffering with mental illness.
- Attachments. Spending time with other professionals such as community psychiatric nurses and social workers is both useful and enlightening. These are the authentic experts.

Reading

Armstrong E (1995) *Mental Health Issues in Primary Care: a practical guide*. Palgrave Macmillan, Basingstoke.

Banks (1994) *Drug Misuse: a practical handbook for the GP.* Blackwell Scientific, London.

Craig T and Davies T (1998) *ABC of Mental Health.* BMJ Books, London.

DOH (1999) *Drug Misuse and Dependence: guidelines on clinical management.* The Stationery Office, London.

Egan G (1994) *The Skilled Helper (5e).* Brooks/Cole Publishing, California.

Gelder M, Gath D, Mayou R and Cowen P (1996) *Oxford Textbook of Psychiatry (3e).* Oxford University Press, Oxford.

Keithley J and Marsh G (1995) *Counseling in Primary Health Care.* Oxford University Press, Oxford.

Kendrick T, Tylee A and Freeling P (1996) *The Prevention of Mental Illness in Primary Care.* Cambridge University Press, Cambridge.

Nelson Jones R (1997) *Practical Counselling and Helping Skills.* Cassell, London.

Ogden J (1996) *Health Psychology: a textbook.* Open University, Buckingham.

Paton A (1994) *ABC of Alcohol (3e).* BMJ Books, London.

Salinsky J and Sackin P (2002) *What Are You Feeling, Doctor?* Radcliffe Medical Press, Oxford.

Skinner R and Cleese J (1993) *Families and How to Survive Them.* Random House, UK.

The Arts

A rich source of insight into mental illness in all its forms. Sources here are too numerous to list but examples might include the books Sylvia Plath's *The Bell Jar* (depression) and Ian McEwen's *Enduring Love* (de Clerambault's syndrome); the films *One Flew over the Cuckoo's Nest* (institutionalisation) and *Shine* (manic depression); and Shakespeare's plays *King Lear* and *Hamlet* (both a fine display of pathological family dynamics and depressive psychoses). You and your trainer can spend a happy afternoon exploring others.

Test yourself

Why do some GPs miss depression?

How do you assess suicidal risk?

What drugs would you choose in a formulary for depression and in a formulary for schizophrenia? What is your justification for this?

What specific issues would you need to consider in arranging a compulsory admission for a patient?

What are the advantages and disadvantages of caring for people with drug addiction by general practitioners as opposed to referral to specialist services?

What strategies do you have for dealing with a patient threatening violence?

Topic 4 Undifferentiated and trivial problems in general practice

In this section an attempt has been made to group together problems that are difficult to classify elsewhere. Included here are day-to-day problems which occur in general practice but are difficult to define in diagnostic terms. These have conventionally been labelled as 'minor' or 'bread and butter' problems. However, the definition of 'minor' depends upon the experience and skill of the doctor and the problem may not be viewed as minor by the patient. What might appear minor at the outset may lead to something more complex or serious, but then again it might not! Differentiating the trivial from the potentially serious is a great challenge. Furthermore, some of these problems may be complex and require a fair degree of diagnostic skill to unravel.

What should be learned

At the end of training, the GP registrar will be able to:

- describe the management of the following miscellaneous symptoms
  - dizziness
  - tiredness all the time
  - significant weight loss conditions
  - significant weight gain and or obesity
  - localised swelling/mass at various sites
  - non-specific rashes
  - allergic problems
  - excessive sweating, localised and generalised
- describe the management of some other problems, e.g. minor respiratory infections, nits, threadworms, aphthous ulcers, scabies, furred tongue, excessive wind, ear wax, verrucas, etc.

- demonstrate an awareness of the concept of presentation due to underlying psychosocial problems or the use of very trivial problems as a passport for entry to see the doctor.

How to do it

- Experiential learning and one-to-one discussion is probably the principal method of learning. Seeing patients, identifying your educational need and discussion with your trainer is likely to be the most beneficial way of addressing this area.
- Follow-up slips. This is a cunning method of following up cases that you have seen. A slip is inserted into the notes of, say, 100 consecutive patients. When the patient sees the next doctor the slip is removed from the notes, comments added and returned to you. Are you missing a hidden agenda? Do the patients you see with 'minor' problems return the next week to disclose child abuse or drug addiction? More details of the 'Follow-up slip system' is to be found at www. londondeanery.ac.uk.

Reading

Fry J and Sandler G (1998) *Common Diseases, their Nature, Incidence and Care (5e)*. Librapharm/Petroc Press, Newbury.

Hopcroft K and Forte V (1999) *Symptom Sorter*. Radcliffe Medical Press, Oxford.

Johnson G, Hill-Smith I and Ellis C (1999) *The Minor Illness Manual*. Radcliffe Medical Press, Oxford.

Knot A and Polmear A (1999) *Practical General Practice*. Butterworth-Heinemann, Oxford.

Stearn M (1998) *Embarrassing Problems*. Health Press, Oxford.

Test yourself

What are the commonest causes of a patient complaining of being 'tired all the time'?

How would you manage a well child with an isolated lump in the neck?

An elderly resident of a nursing home has scabies. How do you manage this?

A young man presents with excessive generalised sweating. How do you decide what to do?

Describe the management of an elderly patient presenting with dizziness?

How would you manage a patient who constantly complains of not being able to lose weight?

Topic 5 Emergencies in general practice

The GP registrar must emerge from a year in general practice competent and confident to deal with a range of emergencies. Clear plans for the management of the common emergencies must be formulated and the appropriate drugs and equipment carried. There is no substitute for experience, but unfortunately emergencies in primary care do not come our way that often. This makes it even more difficult to learn and more importantly, maintain our skills. Remember also that what the patient considers an emergency might not be considered an emergency by us, and vice versa.

What should be learned

At the end of training, the GP registrar will be able to:

- describe management plans for the common emergencies in practice, e.g. myocardial infarction, stroke, status asthmaticus, acute psychosis
- demonstrate competence and confidence when dealing with emergencies
- list and justify the contents of the emergency bag
- demonstrate an understanding of the effects of real or imagined emergencies on patients and their carers
- demonstrate proficiency in basic life support; a certificate attesting to this fact is a necessary pre-requisite for membership of the RCGP
- demonstrate an appropriate use of emergency and out-of-hours services, e.g. accident and emergency department, ambulance, social services.

How to do it

- Observation and experience. Being on call with your trainer at the start of the year enables learning by observation and allows them to assess your ability and confidence in managing primary care emergencies. For a more intensive experience, an attachment to your local out-of-hours co-operative is likely to increase the yield of serious conditions in primary care.

- Clinical attachment. If you were lucky or unlucky enough to miss out on an A&E post during the hospital component of your vocational training then why not consider a few sessions in your local A&E department? They would be very happy to see you.
- A tutorial or tutorials on emergencies at the start of the year is essential. Dealing with emergencies in the home is a very different affair from coping with similar cases in a hospital. You must demonstrate competence before you can take your place in the out-of-hours rota. Your trainer should also cover the contents – and their potential uses – of the doctor's bag at an early stage.
- Skills laboratories and simulators. Most hospitals boast a resuscitation training officer; alternatively, contact your local ambulance unit to find out where their training is carried out. Some teaching hospitals have developed skills laboratories where you can practise emergency medicine without the risk of actually harming anyone.

Reading

Brown A (2002) *Accident and Emergency Diagnosis and Management (4e)*. Arnold Press, London.

Dwight O and Collier J (eds) (2001) *Guidelines for the Management of Common Medical Emergencies in General Practice*. National Patients Access Team, London

Harrington R, Hope S, Watts J and Lawrence N (1996) *Handbook of Emergencies in General Practice (2e)*. Oxford University Press, Oxford.

Mehta DK (ed) *British National Formulary*. BMA and the Royal Pharmaceutical Society of Great Britain, London.

Test yourself

A six-month-old baby has been screaming for some hours. It is now 11.00 pm. How would you assess the situation and what are your management options?

You get a telephone call at 10.00 pm about a man of fifty who has severe pain in the chest. What is your plan of action?

A child of two with fever is rushed to your surgery. She is having a convulsion. How do you assess and treat?

A young man has attacked a neighbour because he thought that he was being affected by thought waves. The police call you. What do you do?

Describe your assessment and management of a young adult with a severe attack of asthma.

A 63-year-old woman presents with acute shortness of breath. Describe your assessment of her.

Topic 6 General medical problems

The GP registrar should come to the general practice training year equipped with a basic understanding of general medical problems. This is not an appropriate environment to have to learn the basics of medicine which should have been acquired in the undergraduate years and in the training posts in hospital. The principal task is to apply the basic knowledge to the diagnosis and management of the problems in the general practice environment. This is difficult because one has to pick out the potentially serious diagnosis from among the mass of undifferentiated presenting problems and one has to do this without aggravating anxieties, reinforcing illness behaviour or using investigations inappropriately. Remember that an unusual illness is more likely to be due to an atypical presentation of a common condition.

The medical conditions in which competence in management should be achieved are too numerous to list but include:

- pneumonia
- bronchitis
- thyrotoxicosis
- irritable bowel syndrome
- ischaemic heart disease
- cardiac failure
- diabetes
- asthma
- polyarthritis
- allergies
- urinary tract infections
- ulcer or non-ulcer dyspepsia
- oesophageal reflux
- transient ischaemic attacks
- migraine
- convulsions.

What should be learned

At the end of training, the GP registrar will be able to:

- state the early, and sometimes atypical, presenting signs and symptoms of the major medical conditions
- describe an effective strategy for investigation of these conditions
- state the indications for referral and justify what he/she proposes to manage personally
- describe and justify management plans for the more common medical problems encountered in general practice
- demonstrate examination skills which are effective and practical in the context of general practice; the GP registrar should be competent in all the major systems, including neurology.

How to do it

- Tutorials linked to experience are probably the best teaching. Basic knowledge is adapted and applied to the general practice environment.
- PUNS and DENS (*see* Chapter 2).
- Lectures and discussion at the half-day release courses. The best learning opportunities occur if the lecturer is engaged in a dialogue and not allowed just to lecture.
- If the assessments reveal particular gaps in knowledge, clinical attachments in outpatients for a few weeks will help to plug them.
- Examinations. The MRCGP and for the brave hearted, the MRCP, are excellent spurs to revision. Past papers may be an effective way of identifying your learning needs.

Reading

There are many heavy tomes available but the *Oxford Handbook* series is probably the best starting point. Don't always accept the expert view. Look at the evidence.

Barton S (ed) (2002) *Clinical Evidence*. BMJ Publishing Group, London.

Longmore JM, Longmore M, Torok E and Wilkinson I (2001) *Oxford Handbook of Clinical Medicine*. Oxford University Press Inc., USA.

You are more likely to get up-to-date information from articles in the medical press. Get into the habit of keeping relevant bits of literature and filing them for easy reference later. The *BMJ* and *Update* are particularly useful. Do not turn up your nose at articles in the 'comics' like *Pulse*, *Doctor* and *GP*, they often contain useful management summaries.

Test yourself

Write a protocol for diagnosing and managing irritable bowel syndrome.

How do investigations help you manage the patient who has lost weight.

In what circumstances, and how, would you manage pneumonia at home?

A 60-year-old man has a relapse of his chronic bronchitis. He is wheezy and has a productive cough. He is a smoker. Outline your management plan.

A 28-year-old woman has mild signs of thyrotoxicosis. Her TSH is low and her T4 is high. How do you manage this? She is married, has one child and uses a sheath for contraception.

A 56-year-old man has an Hb of 10 g/dl and an MCV of 101. How do you investigate further in the context of general practice?

A 30-year-old man presents with 'acid' indigestion. He had a similar attack a year ago. What is your management plan?

A 58-year-old woman presents with a history of a transient dysphasia. How would you set out to establish a diagnosis and how would you manage her?

Topic 7 The management of chronic disease

Continuity of care is cited as one of the strengths of general practice and is regarded as an essential component of care in treating patients with chronic diseases. The burden of responsibility for the effective care of most patients with chronic diseases now rests with the general practitioner, with an increasing movement of patients from secondary into primary care. The principal care of conditions such as diabetes, asthma and chronic obstructive pulmonary disease (COPD) is now delivered in the primary care setting.

What should be learned

At the end of training, the GP registrar will be able to:

- describe the natural history, clinical guidelines and management of common chronic diseases managed in general practice (e.g. asthma, chronic obstructive pulmonary disease, diabetes, hypertension, ischaemic heart disease, epilepsy, thyroid disease, heart failure)
- describe the components of effective chronic disease management in general practice; elements of such care might include
    - criteria for diagnosis of condition
    - identification of cases
    - description of how the care will be delivered, i.e. opportunistically or in a special clinic
    - a clinical protocol representing good, acceptable practice (evidence-based where possible) of the chronic condition
    - a means of evaluating the effectiveness of the care delivered, e.g. clinical audit
    - consideration of how a multiprofessional team may impact on the care given

- describe the components of an integrated care pathway for patients suffering with chronic disease
- describe the personal, psychological, social and financial effects of chronic illness on a patient.

How to do it

- Tutorials. Specific chronic diseases represent good topics for tutorials.
- Observe a chronic disease management clinic in a GP practice.
- Conduct an audit on one aspect of chronic disease management and discuss the findings with your trainer or practice team.

Reading

A good general text is recommended. You may then wish to read up in relation to the specific diseases. Don't forget to review articles in the journals as well as guidelines such as the National Institute for Clinical Excellence (NICE) guidelines: www.nice.org.uk.

Clark M and Kumar P (2002) *Clinical Medicine (5e)*. WB Saunders, Philadelphia.
Hasler J (1996) *The Management of Chronic Disease*. Oxford University Press, Oxford.
McWhinney I (1997) *A Textbook of Family Medicine*. Oxford University Press, Oxford.

Test yourself

What are the advantages and disadvantages of running a diabetes mini clinic?

What would you include in a practice guideline for managing osteoporosis?

What arrangement should there be for the monitoring and repeat prescribing of medication for patients with epilepsy?

Write a practice protocol for managing hypothyroidism.

Design a nurse-led clinic for the ongoing management of patients with COPD.

How might you reduce the incidence of stroke in your practice?

Topic 8 Ear, nose and throat

Ear, nose and throat (ENT) problems are a major part of the workload of the general practitioner but most GP registrars will come to the practice year with little or no experience in this field.

What should be learned

At the end of training, the GP registrar will be able to:

- conduct a thorough examination of the ears, nose and throat using appropriate instruments available in general practice, e.g. tuning fork, otoscope
- understand the natural history of the more common nasal problems seen in children and adults, e.g. catarrh and polyposis, and describe management plans for them
- describe practical plans for the detection and management of deafness, tinnitus and childhood speech and language problems
- describe how to evaluate and manage otalgia
- describe how to evaluate and manage the common sinus, mouth, pharyngeal and laryngeal problems
- describe the indications for and methods of referral for such problems as recurrent tonsillitis, chronic secretory otitis media, deafness in adults and speech problems
- demonstrate appropriate skills in otoscopy, aural toileting, nasal packing and nasal cautery.

How to do it

- Experience. The most important learning method is to see appropriate cases, reflect on your experience and discuss what you have seen and managed with your trainer and your peers. There are no universally accepted management strategies for many of the common ENT problems. A good example is glue ear. You will find that the standard treatment meted out by ENT surgeons tends to be the insertion of grommets, but if you look in the literature you will find that there is considerable doubt about their effectiveness in the short term and complications in the long term. It is important therefore to read, think and debate before accepting the wisdom that may be offered to you.

- Observe your trainer and other partners, although this depends on some ENT interest and expertise residing within the practice.
- A clinical attachment to an ENT specialist for a few sessions is worthwhile, particularly if you have had no previous ENT experience. This is especially helpful for polishing up skills in otoscopy, aural toileting, etc.
- Special courses, particularly those concentrating on ENT issues relevant to general practice. Ask your local primary care tutor if he is aware of any courses available locally.
- Discuss the core ENT subjects at a half-day release session. Why not invite your local ENT consultant along for a question and answer session?

Reading

Textbooks are not likely to be sufficiently up to date or general practice oriented to be of much help with the management of such problems as glue ear, management of sore throats, etc. You are best advised to look out for review articles in the journals, particularly those produced specifically for GPs. Books are more likely to be of help with anatomy and diagnosis.

Browning GG (1994) *Updated ENT (3e)*. Butterworth-Heinemann, Oxford.

Ludman H (1997) *ABC of Otolaryngology*. BMJ Books, London.

Test yourself

Look in an ear with your otoscope. Draw and label a picture of what you see. Check in a textbook. Do you know what you are looking at?

What are your referral criteria for grommet insertion? On what evidence are they based?

A 63-year-old man presents with tinnitus. Describe your management plan?

The parents of an 18-month-old child are concerned about her hearing. How can this be assessed?

Outline the treatment of otitis media in different age groups supporting your answer with current evidence.

A 40-year-old woman presents with multiple small white patches in the mouth. What is the differential diagnosis and how would you manage the problem from here?

Topic 9 Rheumatology and orthopaedics

Musculoskeletal problems are a major part of the workload in general practice and a considerable cause of morbidity and loss of time from work. Undergraduate training in this area is often skimpy and most of the training posts in hospital do not include either rheumatology or orthopaedics. Accident and emergency posts will provide some experience of trauma to muscles, bones and joints. The GP registrar year affords a relatively short time in which to attain a reasonable level of competence in more chronic musculoskeletal conditions.

What should be learned

At the end of training, the GP registrar will be able to:

- demonstrate effective examination of muscles and joints and interpret the signs
- recognise and describe the natural history of common soft tissue and connective tissue disorders, e.g. polymyalgia rheumatica, and to be able to formulate an appropriate management plan and justify any investigations
- recognise and describe the natural history of common joint problems, e.g. osteoarthritis, gout, and be able to formulate an appropriate management plan and justify any investigations
- recognise and describe the natural history of common spinal problems, e.g. back pain, neck pain, and to be able to formulate an appropriate management plan and justify any investigations
- recognise and describe the natural history of common systematic rheumatological problems, e.g. osteoporosis, and to be able to formulate an appropriate management plan and justify any investigations
- understand the role of allied professions, e.g. physiotherapist, osteopath, and refer appropriately

- perform a range of joint and soft tissue injections, e.g. for tennis elbow, frozen shoulder
- recognise and describe the natural history of common childhood orthopaedic, joint and connective tissue disorders.

How to do it

- Observe your trainer and other partners, although this depends on some rheumatological interest and expertise residing within the practice.
- A clinical attachment to a rheumatologist for a few sessions is well worthwhile.
- Special courses, particularly those concentrating on joint injections. Many such courses use simulators which will let you safely get the hang of injections. Once back at the surgery, practise injections on live patients under supervision.
- Spend some time with your local physiotherapist, osteopath or chiropractor. Their knowledge of musculoskeletal anatomy will far surpass yours. It's worth checking out the evidence base for their interventions though.

Reading

Carr A and Harnden A (1995) *Orthopaedics in Primary Care*. Butterworth-Heinemann, Oxford.

Hutson MA (1996) *Sports Injuries: recognition and management (3e)*. Oxford University Press, Oxford.

Silver T (2001) *Joint and Soft Tissue Injection (3e)*. Radcliffe Medical Press, Oxford.

Snaith M (1999) *ABC of Rheumatology (2e)*. BMJ Books, London.

Test yourself

A young man presents with back pain of sudden onset when he bent over to pick up a child. What is likely to be the pathology here? What is the prognosis and how do you manage the problem?

Can you perform an injection for supraspinatus tendonitis?

Describe the investigations you would arrange for a middle-aged woman with mild to moderate polyarthritis.

A young adult presents with pain in the knee. How confident are you that you know how to elicit the appropriate signs and interpret them?

A child of 10 years is brought to you with a limp. What diagnoses do you suspect? On examination there are no definite signs. How do you manage the situation?

How do you diagnose and manage gout in general practice? What is now the most common aetiological factor?

How would you evaluate persistent pain over the greater trochanter of one hip in a woman of 50 years?

Topic 10 Eye problems

Most GP registrars come to their training year with little or no knowledge of ophthalmology. It is a subject poorly covered at medical school and SHOs will have little or no contact with ophthalmological problems in their hospital years. Ophthalmology is therefore one of the most frequently requested subjects for coverage at the half-day release course. Many eye problems do in fact require expert review but there are a number of conditions that can quite easily be managed in primary care by someone that knows what they are doing. There are also some classic pitfalls that we all need to be aware of, such as the acute glaucoma treated as migraine and the patient with a detached retina referred for a routine neurology appointment. By developing a working knowledge of a few common conditions and an awareness of the more serious ones, you should be able to practise both safely and effectively.

What should be learned

At the end of training, the GP registrar will be able to:

- demonstrate appropriate eye examination skills, including fundoscopy through a dilated pupil, the use of fluorescein and testing visual acuity
- demonstrate an ability to diagnose and treat simple eye conditions, e.g. the red eye, loss of vision, eye pain, eyelid disorders
- describe the signs and symptoms which would indicate an ophthalmic emergency
- list the indications for referral
- describe the role of opticians and optometrists
- list the criteria for being placed on and the provisions of the Blind Register.

How to do it

- Clinical attachment. If you lack confidence, the best way to get a lot of exposure to eye problems is to get a clinical attachment for a few days to an ophthalmic unit with an emergency department. In London the best place for this is probably the casualty department of Moorfields Eye Hospital, but many local eye departments run open access clinics where you can see first presentations of the common eye problems.
- Half-day release. Invite your local ophthalmologist along to talk to you, but make sure the afternoon covers the common primary care problems. He or she will probably have a laptop full of slides which will be useful for diagnostic practice.

Reading

Books with plenty of colour illustrations are best.

Finlay RD and Payne PAG (1997) *The Eye in General Practice (10e)*. Butterworth-Heinemann, Oxford.

Khaw PT (1999) *ABC of Eyes*. BMJ Books, London.

Okhravi N (1997) *Manual of Primary Eye Care*. Butterworth-Heinemann, Oxford.

Test yourself

What are the causes of chronic visual loss? Describe their diagnosis and management.

When would you refer a patient with cataract?

How do you manage a baby with a blocked tear duct?

Can you remove a foreign body from the cornea?

What are the warning signs that a patient might have a detached retina?

A 50-year-old man has a unilateral red eye. How would you assess him?

What are the DVLA regulations relating to reduced vision?

Topic 11 Women's health

If you have undertaken an obstetrics and gynaecology SHO job then you will start here with an advantage, especially if the post included plenty of antenatal and outpatient work. Ideally, you will have already attended a family planning theory course and may also have obtained the Diploma of the Royal College of Obstetricians and Gynaecologists. If not, then you will have another chunk of learning to fit in to an already crowded year.

What should be learned

At the end of training, the GP registrar will be able to:

- examine the female pelvis, recognising normal architecture and common abnormalities
- demonstrate the taking of a competent gynaecological history and an awareness of how psychosexual problems may present
- describe management plans for the common gynaecological disorders, including dysfunctional uterine bleeding, vaginal discharge and premenstrual tension
- list the usual methods of contraception and their indications and contraindications
- describe a management plan for patients requesting a termination of pregnancy
- list the indications for and the benefits of hormone replacement therapy
- describe management plans for patients who complain of infertility
- demonstrate willingness and the ability to give pre-conceptual counselling
- demonstrate an understanding of routine antenatal care, recognise the common problems that present and describe the circumstances under which referral to secondary care would be necessary

- describe a management plan for a patient presenting with a breast lump.

How to do it

- Clinical skills training. Learning about pelvic examination can be done while sitting in with the trainer but the yield of suitable cases is likely to be low. The practice nurse may run a smear clinic, and this would be the ideal environment to hone your speculum skills. Sitting in on a few gynaecology outpatient clinics would also be useful, as unbelievably, some SHOs still do not manage to attend any during their obstetrics and gynaecology posting. Fitting IUCDs and caps is an optional skill and one for which it is mandatory, but often extremely difficult, to arrange training. Ask your trainer and/or course organiser about local arrangements. Apply early for a place as there is often a long waiting list for training.
- Theoretical family planning courses. There are often special courses in family planning. In London, the best known ones are those run by the Margaret Pyke centre.
- Discussion and random case analysis will provide many opportunities to tease out common management problems in gynaecology.

Reading

Anthony J and Kaye P (2001) *Notes for the DRCOG (4e)*. Churchill Livingstone, Oxford.

Guillibaud J (1997) *The Pill and Other Forms of Hormonal Contraception*. Oxford Paperbacks, Oxford.

Guillibaud J (1999) *Contraception: your questions answered*. Churchill Livingstone, Oxford.

McPherson A and Waller D (1997) *Women's Health (4e)*. Oxford University Press, Oxford.

Test yourself

How do you assess and manage a 14-year-old girl with a persistent vaginal discharge?

A 30-year-old married woman complains of symptoms suggestive of premenstrual syndrome. Outline your management.

What is your management plan for a 40-year-old woman with menorrhagia, normal cycle and a slightly bulky uterus?

A young nulliparous woman asks you to fit an IUCD because she cannot remember to take the contraceptive pill regularly. How do you advise her?

What issues will you discuss with a woman asking for advice about whether to start hormone replacement therapy?

You find sugar in the urine of a pregnant woman at 20 weeks gestation. Describe your assessment of her.

What investigations would you perform in the management of an infertile couple?

Describe your management of a pregnant woman with a blood pressure of 145/90: at 12 weeks, at 28 weeks, at 38 weeks?

Topic 12 The care of babies and young children

The richness of general practice is particularly highlighted by the care of babies and young children. The assessment of small children in a general practice setting can be difficult, and any consultation with a child will also include addressing the concerns of the parent or guardian, which poses significant challenges in itself. In addition to clinical knowledge, developing good assessment skills is essential. This is vital because of the overriding need to identify a 'sick' child or child at risk, from a large proportion of generally well children with self-limiting illness. Understanding child developmental issues, and being clear who to refer to, and when, makes this essential area of general practice hugely challenging, but very stimulating.

What should be learned

At the end of training, the GP registrar will be able to:

- describe the main conditions that can be screened for prenatally
- outline the common neonatal problems encountered in general practice and describe strategies for managing them
- describe the normal feeding requirements of babies and the management of common feeding problems
- list the principal developmental milestones and describe strategies for the management of delayed development
- outline the key requirements of a child health surveillance programme
- demonstrate an understanding of how illnesses present in children
- describe management plans for the common childhood illnesses and emergencies
- demonstrate the clinical skills needed for assessing children

- describe the immunisation schedule for children, and the relative and absolute contraindications of vaccines used
- describe the management of common behaviour problems in children
- list the clinical features of child abuse and describe the local arrangements for child protection.

How to do it

- Experience. It is vital to see and assess as many children as possible within the context of general practice both in routine surgeries, in 'emergency' clinics or as part of the 'out of hours' service used by your practice. Dealing with lots of normal children makes it easier to identify an ill child.
- Direct observation of health visitors including attendance at the practice and community child health surveillance clinics.
- Courses. There are a number of regional and national courses on child health promotion and behavioural problems.

Reading

Goldman A (1994) *Care of the Dying Child*. Oxford University Press, Oxford.

Hall D, Hill P and Ellman D (1994) *The Child Surveillance Handbook*. Radcliffe Medical Press, Oxford.

Hall D (1996) *Health For All Children*. Oxford University Press, Oxford.

Hull D and Johnston D (1993) *Essential Paediatrics*. Churchill Livingstone, Edinburgh.

Illingworth R (1991) *The Normal Child*. Churchill Livingstone, Edinburgh.

Modell M, Mughal Z and Boyd R (1996) *Paediatric Problems in General Practice*. Oxford University Press, Oxford.

Valman H (1993) *ABC of One to Seven*. BMJ Books, London.

Test yourself

Describe your management of a 3-month-old baby who is 'failing to thrive'.

How do you assess a baby of four months with a fever of 39°C?

A mother presents with her 20-month-old child who is unable to walk as yet. Describe your management.

A 12-year-old patient is allegedly constantly disruptive at school. How would you assess this situation?

What are the arguments for and against MMR immunisation?

The practice nurse has noted a smelly vaginal discharge in a 7-year-old girl. She is concerned that this may be a case of sexual abuse. Describe your management.

Topic 13 Sexual medicine

Sex plays a significant part in dictating human behaviour and when there are problems there can be significant physical, psychological and relationship consequences. It is often difficult for both patients and doctors to discuss these problems openly. If a doctor is to be able to help patients with such problems he or she must be aware of his or her attitudes to sex and sexuality and be able to discuss sexual problems without embarrassment.

What should be learned

At the end of training, the GP registrar will be able to:

- discuss his/her own attitudes to sex and sexuality
- list common sexual myths
- describe the anatomy and physiology of the human sexual response
- demonstrate how to take a sexual history from a patient
- describe how to formulate a sexual problem in terms of:
  - predisposing factors
  - precipitating factors
  - perpetuating factors
- list the common sexual dysfunctions that may present in general practice and outline the management of these in both psychological terms and physical terms
- describe the epidemiology, natural history and management of the common sexually transmitted diseases prevalent in society
- demonstrate appropriate skills when counselling patients requesting HIV tests or tests for other sexually transmitted diseases
- describe the ethical implications of caring for patients known to have HIV infection or other sexually transmitted diseases.

How to do it

- Small groups. Discussion of attitudes to sex and sexuality as well as psychosexual problems often occurs on the day-release course of the local VTS. Some schemes run specific courses on the management of psychosexual problems.
- Case discussion and tutorials. Regular case reviews can often reveal a potential psychosexual problem, which can then be discussed more fully with your trainer.
- A visit to your local genitourinary medicine clinic may help to clarify what can be tackled in the practice and what should be referred.

Reading

Adler M (1993) *ABC of AIDS (4e)*. BMJ Books, London.
Adler M (1998) *ABC of Sexually Transmitted Disease (5e)*. BMJ Books, London.
Bancroft J (1989) *Human Sexuality and its Problems (2e)*. Churchill Livingstone, Edinburgh.
Carter Y, Moss C and Weyman A (1997) *RCGP Handbook of Sexual Health in Primary Care*. Royal College of General Practitioners, London.
Skrine R (1997) *Blocks and Freedoms in Sexual Life: a handbook of psychosexual medicine*. Radcliffe Medical Press, Oxford.

Test yourself

A 30-year-old homosexual man presents with erectile dysfunction.
Outline your management plan.

Describe the management of vaginismus.

How would you organise a programme for *Chlamydia* screening in
general practice?

What issues would you discuss with a recently pregnant woman
requesting an HIV test?

How might you manage a married man presenting with premature
ejaculation?

Write a practice protocol for the management of genital herpes.

Topic 14 Skin problems in general practice

Skin problems supply a large proportion of the diagnostic uncertainty generated in general practice. GP registrars may come into practice with little relevant dermatological experience and often cite this as an area of great need. Reassuringly most skin problems are harmless, although a few lesions could be markers of a serious disease.

What should be learned

At the end of training, the GP registrar will be able to:

- recognise the common skin complaints prevalent in general practice and describe management plans for them
- describe the features of dermatological lesions that may indicate malignancy and outline a management plan, including indications for referral
- describe a basic formulary for medications that he/she will use in treating common skin complaints and justify the preparations chosen
- describe the skin conditions that may be markers of systemic disease
- outline the practical considerations in setting up a minor surgery service in general practice, to include issues such as consent
- demonstrate practical skills in minor surgery, e.g. the use of cryotherapy, taking of skin scrapings for mycology and histology.

How to do it

- Experience. A significant amount of dermatology experience may be gained simply by repeated exposure to common skin problems presenting in general practice. Make sure you ask your trainer or other partners to have a look if you are not sure about a diagnosis, and encourage them to call you if they see interesting skin problems in their surgeries. Attend your practice's minor surgery clinics to gain practical experience.

- Visits. Your experience can be extended considerably by attending a few dermatology outpatient sessions at your local trust, especially those involving minor surgery and/or cryotherapy.

Reading

A good atlas of dermatology is a vital reference. The Du Vivier book is an excellent example.

Buxton P (1998) *ABC of Dermatology (3e)*. BMJ Books, London.

Du Vivier A (2002) *Atlas of Clinical Dermatology (3e)*. Churchill Livingstone, Edinburgh.

Hunter J, Savin J and Dahl M (1994) *Clinical Dermatology*. Blackwell, Oxford.

Kneebone R and Schofield J (1998) *Minor Surgery and Skin Lesions, CD-ROM*. Royal College of General Practitioners, London.

Stuart Brown J (2001) *Minor Surgery: a text and atlas (3e)*. Arnold, London.

Test yourself

Discuss your management of an 18-year-old girl recently diagnosed with psoriasis.

What would you write into a practice guideline for the treatment of acne?

What are the indications for referral of pigmented skin lesions?

Write a protocol for setting up a minor surgery service in general practice.

Develop a section of a practice formulary for the treatment of eczema.

List the infectivity and exclusion periods for the common childhood rashes.

Topic 15 Care of the elderly

The care of the elderly has always contributed a major part of the workload of any general practice. Elderly patients often have multiple problems as a result of a multisystem failure. A significant proportion of the elderly are on multiple medications and caring for the elderly truly relies on a multidisciplinary approach and an integrated care pathway. Increasingly, caring for the elderly is becoming a local and national priority and the recent *National Service Framework* (NSF) in elderly care has highlighted specific priorities, some of which will have considerable implications for general practice in terms of time and workload.

What should be learned

At the end of training, the GP registrar will be able to:

- describe the consequences of the normal ageing process on physical, psychological and social wellbeing
- define the terms impairment, disability and handicap as applied to the elderly
- describe the management of some common problems that affect the elderly
  - falls
  - hypothermia
  - dementia
  - parkinsonism
- describe the particular problems of prescribing for the elderly
- describe the roles of members of the primary healthcare team and other agencies who may be involved in the care of the elderly

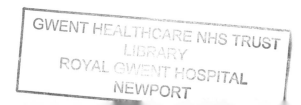

- outline the local support services for the elderly in your locality including those provided by the local authority and voluntary organisations
- describe the different types of residential care accommodation in your area and the criteria used to decide placement within them.

How to do it

- Experience. Ensure that you get adequate exposure to caring for elderly patients. You may wish to discuss with your trainer ways of building up a suitable case mix.
- Visits. Home visits as well as visits to nursing homes will provide valuable experience. You may wish to accompany your trainer on follow-up visits to elderly patients. Another good way to gain experience is accompanying a geriatrician on domiciliary visits to your practice's patients. You may also wish to visit your local elderly day hospital and sit in on some outpatient clinics.

Reading

Coni N, Davison W and Webster S (1992) *Ageing: the facts (2e)*. Oxford University Press, Oxford.

Department of Health (2002) *National Service Framework for Elderly Care*. DoH, London.

Grimsley Evans J and Franklin WT (1992) *Oxford Textbook of Geriatric Medicine*. Oxford University Press, Oxford.

Idris Williams E (1995) *Caring for Older People in the Community*. Radcliffe Medical Press, Oxford.

Sidell M (1995) *Health in Old Age: myth, mystery and management*. Oxford University Press, Oxford.

Test yourself

What is the value of regular health checks for the elderly?

What would you put into a 'guideline' for preventing falls in the elderly to be used by district nurses?

Describe how you would assess a confused elderly patient living alone at home.

How would you go about admitting an elderly patient into respite accommodation?

The wife of a 78-year-old man complains that her husband is becoming forgetful. Describe your management.

Write a section for a practice formulary on Parkinson's disease.

Topic 16 Terminal care and bereavement

During the course of the training year, the average GP registrar is unlikely to see a patient right through the terminal phase of a serious illness. This is due to a number of interrelated factors; experience, case load, duration of time in the practice, the need for a patient and family to have a familiar face around at a difficult time and so on. However, even if one of your own patients does not require terminal care at home, there is no reason why you should not assist with one of your trainer's, or with a patient of another partner in the practice. Dealing with death, dying and bereavement is an important and difficult part of our work and will challenge your own personal resources as well as making you realise how much better things can be if these are pooled with the thoughts, feelings and skills of others. Terminal care is the multiprofessional discipline *par excellence*.

What should be learned

At the end of training, the GP registrar will be able to:

- demonstrate an understanding of the normal process of bereavement across all ages and cultural boundaries
- understand the abnormalities of grieving that may occur and outline their predisposing factors
- list the professionals and the agencies that may be able to help the bereaved
- demonstrate an understanding of what constitutes good terminal care
- describe management plans for the control of pain and for the other main symptoms of the dying such as vomiting, constipation or hiccups
- list the dosages, methods of administration and side-effects of the drugs used

- demonstrate an ability to prepare individuals and their families for death
- understand the processes and protocols governing death and cremation, certification, and the role of the coroner.

How to do it

- Experience. The most important learning method is to see appropriate cases, reflect on your experience and discuss what you have seen and managed with your trainer and your peers. Make sure that early in the year your trainer puts you into contact with patients who may become terminally ill. You can then establish a relationship and undertake their terminal care under the guidance of your trainer.
- Hospice visits. Make contact with the medical director of your local hospice. Most will be overjoyed to see you and keen to teach. The outreach workers or Macmillan nurses will likewise be more than happy to take you on their rounds and it is from them that you will learn how to manage the common symptoms of the terminal patient.
- Special courses, particularly those concentrating on the medical management of terminal care or communication skills with the bereaved. Ask your local hospice medical director or primary care tutor if he or she is aware of any courses available locally.
- Discuss patients you have found difficult to manage at the half-day release session.

Reading

There are a few classic books which you should read but perhaps more powerfully, films, novels and the theatre can provide deep insights into these universal experiences (*see* The Arts).

Doyle D (1994) *Domiciliary Palliative Care: a handbook for family doctors and community nurses.* Oxford University Press, Oxford.

Kubler-Ross E (1973) *On Death and Dying.* Routlege, London.

Parkes CM (1998) *Bereavement: studies of grief in adult life (3e).* Penguin, London.

The Arts

Experiences of death, dying and bereavement can be found illuminated in many books, plays, films and poems. Here are one or two examples. You will also have your own.

Bennett A (1982) *A Woman of No Importance.* Samuel French, London.

Dunn D (1985) *Elegies.* Faber and Faber, London.

Lewis CS (1961) *A Grief Observed.* Faber and Faber, London.

Truly, Madly, Deeply (1990) dir. Minghella.

Test yourself

A woman is still very disturbed a year after her husband's death. How do you assess and manage the problem?

A man who is dying of carcinoma of the prostate does not want to go into a hospice. What help can you get for him and his wife?

How do you obtain and set up a syringe driver at home?

What particular problems do you face when managing a dying child?

An elderly woman has just been diagnosed as having terminal carcinoma of the cervix. Her husband comes to see you to ask that she is not told about the diagnosis. How do you handle this situation?

An 85-year-old man dies in his sleep at home having not seen a doctor for three months. What arrangements need to be made regarding death certification?

Topic 17 Preventive medicine and immunisation

Preventive medicine has become an increasingly important aspect of general practice. The health economic argument is strongly in favour of prevention versus cure and for several years the performance of GPs has been measured by how effective they are at reaching prevention targets. Such activities may be delegated to other members of the practice team, but ultimately the responsibility rests with the GP.

What should be learned

At the end of training, the GP registrar will be able to:

- define what is meant by the terms primary, secondary and tertiary prevention
- state the scientific principles of screening and describe some criteria that make for an effective screening programme
- outline the screening methods that may be used in general practice and state the advantages and disadvantages of each, e.g. case finding versus population screening
- describe the current epidemiology of diseases for which screening programmes or other preventive measures may be worthwhile within the context of general practice
- demonstrate that he/she can deliver preventive measures within a consultation where it is appropriate to do so
- describe the roles of other primary healthcare team members in the delivery of preventive care
- outline how to set up a screening or other preventive programme in primary care
- describe current immunisation schedules for adults, including those for particular professions

- describe specific measures to prevent illness in people travelling overseas.

How to do it

- Observation. Identify how your training practice organises preventive work. You should find out how immunisations are organised, gain experience of preventive clinics and also discuss the roles other members of the practice team have in delivering preventive healthcare.
- Visits. You should visit other practices during your training and gain experience of how other practices organise preventive healthcare. A visit to the local Director of Public Health may also be of benefit. Public health directors may be contacted through your local primary care trust.
- Project work. This is a fertile area for project work or audit. You may wish to focus on a particular area of preventive care and evaluate its effectiveness.

Reading

Austoker J (1995) *Cancer Prevention in Primary Care*. BMJ Books, London.

Department of Health (1996) *Immunisation against Infectious Disease*. The Stationery Office, London.

Fowler G, Muir Gray J and Anderson P (1993) *Prevention in General Practice*. Oxford University Press, Oxford.

Naidoo J and Willis J (1994) *Health Promotion: foundations for practice*. Balliere Tindall, London.

Walker E, Williams G and Raeside F (1997) *ABC of Health Travel*. BMJ Books, London.

Test yourself

What are the arguments for and against screening for prostate cancer?

What factors would you consider in deciding whether to set up a programme for glaucoma screening in general practice?

What roles do your practice nurse and health visitor play in screening programmes within your practice?

What health education methods can be used in general practice? Discuss their effectiveness.

What health advice would you give to a 28-week pregnant woman who wishes to fly to the Gambia?

Write an evidence-based protocol for the use of pneumococcal vaccine within the practice.

Topic 18 Prescribing

Prescribing is what we do all day. We give a small slip of green paper to two thirds of the people that enter and leave our office. Prescribing is the action in our action plan, and therefore essential to perform appropriately and safely. Prescribing is also an expensive activity; over £6 billion is spent by the NHS on prescriptions each year – a figure which continues to grow by around 10% per year. As a result, prescribing must also be carried out with a wary eye to cost and effectiveness.

What should be learned

At the end of training, the GP registrar will be able to:

- prescribe rationally and precisely, including controlled drugs, with due attention to regulation and cost
- prescribe safely demonstrating an awareness of important drug contraindications, adverse effects, interactions and the need for monitoring
- evaluate and where necessary act on, published evidence and guidance, including that of the National Institute of Clinical Excellence (NICE), about the appropriateness of specific treatments
- appreciate the principles of appropriate repeat prescribing
- interpret prescribing data, including prescribing and practice activity (PACT), and understand how it may be used to improve practice
- produce an audit(s) of prescribing behaviour in the practice
- demonstrate an awareness of prescribing procedures for patients with special needs, e.g. drug addicts, patients in nursing homes, patients requiring domiciliary oxygen
- appreciate the factors that affect patient compliance.

How to do it

- Attach yourself to your local community pharmacist. Question anything you don't understand. The primary care trust will also employ a prescribing adviser who may be able to take you on one of her practice visits.
- PACT data. What are the top 20 cost drugs in your practice? Why? What percentage of drugs is prescribed generically? You can also obtain PACT data on your own prescribing by annotating your prescriptions.
- Audit. Computerisation makes audits of prescribing quick and easy.
- Random case analysis. Compare your prescribing with your trainers.
- Project. Produce a chapter for the practice formulary or write a protocol for the use of a specific drug.

Reading

Most books on prescribing will be out of date as soon as they are written. The following regular publications are therefore the most useful references around.

British National Formulary: This is an amazing book and probably the most useful reference you will ever come across in your career. The first 30 pages or so are packed with useful information relating to all matters pertaining to prescribing, from drugs allowed in sport to prescribing in terminal care. The *BNF* is distributed free to all GP registrars, or should be, every six months.

Drug and Therapeutics Bulletin: An independent monthly publication circulated to all GPs by the Consumers' Association, the publishers of *Which?*, the *DT&B* will usually get around to reviewing the majority of new therapeutic developments.

National Institute of Clinical Excellence Guidance: Now published regularly in a handy compilation form, *NICE Guidance* will help you in negotiations with patients about such thorny issues as weight-reducing medication, and interferon for multiple sclerosis.

Clinical Evidence: Not just a prescribing resource but a summary of all the quality evidence relating to specific interventions. Each chapter divides interventions into 'beneficial', 'likely to be beneficial', 'unknown effectiveness' and 'likely to be ineffective or harmful'. A condensed summary version is now published and disseminated to all practices. *Clinical Evidence* is also available on line via the National electronic Library for Health (NeLH), which is useful as each successive complete volume gets exponentially heavier.

Test yourself

Name your top three choices of NSAIDs. List the criteria you used for making your choice.

How will you audit your repeat prescribing system in your practice? List your criteria.

What are your indications for the use of proton pump inhibitors?

Produce the chapter on cardiovascular drugs for a practice formulary.

An obese mature onset diabetic needs treatment. What drug or drugs would you use? Justify your choice.

How would you best prescribe methadone for an opiate addict?

Write an evidence-based review on the selection of antidepressants in primary care.

What are the pros and cons of speaking to drug company representatives?

Topic 19 Management and finance in general practice

The management and fiscal aspects of general practice are much neglected during training, yet surveys of young principals all show that they would have liked to have learned much more about these subjects during their registrar year. Management and finance can be a big turn off in the registrar year. This has much to do with the immediacy of application of other more clinically based skills and knowledge, and a corresponding perceived irrelevance of financial and managerial matters. Remind yourself that in a few months you may be responsible for organising a practice and employing staff!

What should be learned

At the end of training, the GP registrar will be able to:

- describe the roles of all the members of the practice team
- state the responsibilities of an employer and the basics of employment law as it applies to general practice
- describe the management structure of the practice, how decisions are made and how responsibilities are shared or delegated
- demonstrate a working knowledge of the Terms of Service and the Statement of Fees and Allowances
- demonstrate the ability to be an effective member, or leader of a team
- understand the importance of team dynamics in the functioning of an organisation
- demonstrate an ability to delegate effectively
- describe the basic accounting systems that are needed for the running of a general practice

- describe how the various functions of the practice are organised and administered, e.g. appointment systems, repeat prescribing, clinics, the taking of visits, etc.
- demonstrate an understanding of how the practice functions as a business and the implications various activities and expenses have on the profitability
- describe how staff should be selected, motivated and managed
- describe the methods used for staff development including education, training, appraisal, etc.
- advertise for, and interview new practice staff in accordance with the law and principles relating to equal opportunities
- demonstrate an understanding of how partnerships function and of the importance of good partnership agreements
- describe strategies for communicating effectively within the organisation and with other organisations
- describe the process of, and factors that influence, change
- describe the process of drawing up a practice development plan
- describe alternative systems of healthcare delivery to that provided by the training practice.

How to do it

- Observation. Arrange one-to-one sessions with all the various members of the practice team to grasp just what it is that they do and how they contribute to the business. Do this early on in the year and then go back and clarify issues as they become more important to you.
- Tutorials. These are usually from the partner most interested in management (often not your trainer) or from the practice manager.
- Practice visits. Find out how other practices work. In particular, visit practices that are different from your own: single handed, PMS practices, etc.

- Accountant. It is well worth getting to know the practice accountant, although this can come at a price. Usually the accountant will visit the practice to discuss an annual financial report. Make sure you attend this meeting and go through the accounts with someone who knows what they are talking about.
- Meetings. Practices generally hold a number of different types of meetings ranging from away-days to discuss the practice development plan to day-to-day business meetings to discuss the colour of the doormat. Make sure you are invited to all of these and contribute where appropriate.
- Projects. A management project is the best way to force yourself to learn. Take on the responsibility for some aspect of management in the practice and all the problems will suddenly become apparent!

Reading

Belbin R (1981) *Management Teams: why they succeed or fail.* Heinemann Professional Publishing, Oxford.

Bogle I (2002) *Succeeding as a General Practitioner: the experts share their secrets.* Health Press, Oxford.

Bogle I, Chisholm J and Ellis N (1997) *Making Sense of the Red Book.* Radcliffe Medical Press, Oxford.

Chisholm J, Ellis N and Lawrence-Parr C (1998) *General Practice Employment Handbook.* Radcliffe Medical Press, Oxford.

Dean J (2000) *Making Sense of Practice Finance.* Radcliffe Medical Press, Oxford.

Elwyn G, Greenhalgh T and Macfarlane F (2001) *Groups: a guide to small group work in healthcare, management, education and research.* Radcliffe Medical Press, Oxford.

Irvine S and Haman H (1997) *Making Sense of Personnel Management.* Radcliffe Medical Press, Oxford.

Jay A (1976) How to Run a Meeting. Booklet to accompany the film *'Meetings, Bloody Meetings'.* Video Arts, London.

Pringle M (1993) *Change and Teamwork in Primary Care.* BMJ Books, London.

Pritchard P and Pritchard J (1992) *Developing Teamwork in Primary Health Care.* Oxford Medical Publications, Oxford.

The Journals *Medeconomics* and *Financial Pulse* are also well worth scanning. They are usually full of quite useful tips.

Test yourself

The appointment system is not working well. The doctors are booked up three or more days in advance and the receptionists are under pressure from the patients. How do you set about reviewing the system?

One receptionist is often away sick for minor illness and she is often inappropriately bad tempered with patients. How do you set about managing this problem?

The practice profits fell last year. How do you analyse the situation? What remedies may be offered?

You are going to employ a new practice manager. Write a job description and a contract of employment.

The partners spend a long time every morning on what seems to be a disproportionately large number of repeat prescriptions. What could be done to improve the situation?

What precautions can partners take to minimise the risks of partnership disputes?

Describe a training programme for the new receptionist.

Nurse-led triage is soon to be introduced into your practice. What strategies can you think of for managing that change effectively?

What makes a practice meeting effective?

What methods does your practice use to communicate information within the organisation? What are the advantages and disadvantages of the methods used?

Topic 20 The organisation of healthcare

The organisation of healthcare may not appear immediately relevant to your training but will undoubtedly have relevance once training is completed and a career in general practice unfolds. Healthcare is constantly changing and within the past five years primary care has been reorganised many times and the changes are likely to continue.

What should be learned

At the end of training, the GP registrar will be able to:

- describe the management structure of the NHS (this week!)
- list the main agencies involved in delivering healthcare including local authority agencies, alternative providers, private sector and ancillary sources of primary care, e.g. NHS Direct, 'walk-in centres', etc.
- outline how the organisations delivering healthcare are monitored
- describe the means by which general practice is represented politically.

How to do it

- Tutorials. Probably the best way for understanding how the health service is organised locally. Small groups on the VTS day-release course will allow understanding of your role within a group and give some experience of group dynamics.
- Visits. Visits to your local medical committee (LMC) and to public meetings of your PCT or health authority can be helpful to understand the local political issues.

Reading

Unfortunately no textbook can keep up with the pace of change in the NHS. It is probably better to survey the journals and medical newspapers for up-to-date information.

Boyd R (1996) *What is the Future for a Primary Care-led NHS?* Radcliffe Medical Press, Oxford.

Test yourself

Construct a chart demonstrating the NHS organisations within your locality and how they relate to each other.

What are the roles of the Strategic Health Authority, Workforce Development Confederation and the PCT?

How are GPs represented politically?

What are the local health priorities for your PCT?

What are the functions of the LMC?

How are the views of GPs represented politically at a local and national level?

What are the benefits to the PCT of developing GPs with special interests?

Topic 21 Audit, quality and clinical governance

The ability to critically reflect on and refine our performance, both personal and clinical, is an important life skill. At the level of patient care, the healthy scepticism engendered by an evidence-based approach to healthcare is a feisty alternative to being fed your lines by experts, encouraging, as it does, a reiterative questioning of our own clinical practice. But 'what we do' is only part of the story, and 'who we are' and 'how we do it' may be every bit as important from the patient's perspective. Reflective practice, audit and patient feedback are all important and improving influences but, as if that wasn't enough, the Government would also like us to do it better, through appraisal, clinical governance and quality initiatives.

What should be learned

At the end of training, the GP registrar will be able to:

- produce at least one complete audit cycle – a requirement of summative assessment (SA) – and describe the processes involved, both of the audit itself and in achieving change within the practice
- demonstrate the ability to critically appraise his or her strengths and weaknesses as a GP
- understand the principles of clinical governance and how these apply to his/her practice
- demonstrate an awareness of the systems for monitoring standards of care in the UK
- understand and apply critical appraisal skills and other techniques used in the practice of evidence-based healthcare
- demonstrate the ability to elicit and respond appropriately to feedback from patients and colleagues

- demonstrate an awareness of national quality initiatives, e.g. those organised through the RCGP
- write a personal development plan (PDP)
- appreciate the importance of a whole practice approach to the improvement of patient care.

How to do it

- A completed audit cycle is the most common method adopted for satisfying the written submission component of SA. Hopefully this will not be the only audit that you carry out during the training year. Audit is a powerful tool for change and one which will play an important role throughout the rest of your career.
- Ask. *See* Feedback from patients, staff and colleagues in Chapter 2.
- Reflective practice through case analysis. Richard Eve's PUNs and DENs (*see* Chapter 2) is a useful starting point for clinical introspection, although any process that encourages reflective thought about actual patient encounters will result in real learning.
- Evidence-based medicine and critical appraisal courses. It is quite likely that your trainer will not feel very confident about teaching you critical appraisal, although they will probably know more than they think they do. Courses on critical appraisal are run throughout the country, although we would recommend that you book onto one that will teach you sustainable skills rather than just as a crammer for the MRCGP examination.
- Set up and undergo a series of appraisals with your trainer. What does it feel like? How would you have done it better?
- Spend some time with the clinical governance lead of your local PCT. It's a lonely job; they will be pleased to have some company.

Reading

Greenhalgh T (1997) *How to Read a Paper.* BMJ Books, London.

Guyatt G and Drummond R (2002) *Users' Guides to the Medical Literature.* AMA Press, Chicago.

Mulligan J (1988) *The Personal Management Handbook: how to make the most of your potential.* Sphere, London.

Rughani A (2000) *The GP's Guide to Personal Development Plans.* Radcliffe Medical Press, Oxford.

Test yourself

Next time a patient presents you with a clipping from the *Daily Mail* extolling the benefits of a new wonder cure, search out and critically appraise the available evidence.

Design, and use, a patient feedback questionnaire.

Analyse the *doctor's educational needs* (DENs) of your next 20 patients.

Design an audit looking at some non-clinical aspect of your training practice.

What information is your training practice required to submit to the PCT as part of the local clinical governance programme?

What is the difference between appraisal and performance review?

Develop a practice initiative to improve the quality of care to patients within the locality.

Topic 22 Ethics, probity and the law

These areas have become increasingly prominent in modern day practice, as a greater awareness of the ethical issues under-pinning the work of a GP has emerged. It is worth remembering that medical ethics help doctors understand what is right and wrong in medicine, and medical law examines what is lawful medicine. Therefore a GP needs to understand the legal frame-work of any particular medical issue, and also the various ethical frameworks too. Ethical reasoning helps in identifying the 'right' decision but is more important in justifying the decision.

What should be learned

At the end of training, the GP registrar will be able to:

- recognise and explore ethical issues arising in general practice
- apply a framework for ethical reasoning when confronted with ethical dilemmas arising in general practice
- describe the professional responsibilities of a doctor as defined by the General Medical Council (GMC)
- describe the legal frameworks that underpin the work of a doctor.

How to do it

- Tutorials and case discussion. Sharing ethical problems and discussing them with colleagues is the most relevant way of learning. Tutorials with your trainer and small group discussion on the VTS half-day release course are excellent opportunities to explore ethical problems.
- Modified essay questions. Past papers from the MRCGP examination provide plenty of discussion material and

recent questions have explored issues as diverse as euthanasia, patient representation and paternity testing.

Reading

Beauchamp T and Childress J (2001) *Principles of Biomedical Ethics (5e)*. Oxford University Press, Oxford.

Essex B (1994) *Doctors, Dilemmas, Decisions*. BMJ Books, London.

General Medical Council (2001) *Good Medical Practice (3e)*, GMC, London.

Gillon R (1986) *Philosophical Medical Ethics*. John Wiley and Sons, Chichester.

Pickersgill D (1992) *The Law and General Practice*. Radcliffe Medical Press, Oxford.

Royal College of General Practitioners and the General Practitioner Committee of the BMA (2002) *Good Medical Practice for General Practitioners*, RCGP, London.

Toon P (1999) *Towards a Philosophy of General Practice: a study of the virtuous practitioner*. Occasional Paper No. 78. Royal College of General Practitioners, London.

Test yourself

When is consent truly 'informed'?

An HGV driver has recently been diagnosed with epilepsy and continues to drive. What would you do?

One of your medical colleagues has been noted to be drinking heavily before commencing his surgery. How do you decide what to do?

Should patients have to pay for home visits? What ethical principles inform your decision?

Would you/should you accept a Christmas gift of £50 from a patient?

What safeguards exist within your practice to prevent financial fraud?

7

Reading for the registrar year

How to read

We have all had that experience of revising for an examination and being unable to remember anything that we read the night before. The usual reason for such amnesia – well, the non-alcohol-related reason anyway – is that we just don't retain information that isn't useful to us. A blanket approach to reading doesn't work.

As we've seen, adults learn best by experience. Experience makes us aware of our areas of weakness, highlighting our learning needs. If we catch these learning needs before they are drowned out by the next batch, we can develop, grow and learn. If we don't, the gap is covered over by aberrant coping strategies and the impetus to improve is lost. Adults learn most effectively when there is immediacy of application, i.e. the thing you read today is put into practice tomorrow. So make your reading relevant, read when you need to know, when a particular patient raises a particular question in your mind, and make it immediate, don't leave finding out until the next day; *Carpe diem*.

Such is the pace of change in primary care that much of what you will need to know cannot be found in books. Again, indiscriminate browsing of journals, although occasionally entertaining, is an ineffective learning strategy. As David Sackett points out, there are many more reasons for writing an article than there are for reading one! Small group learning is an efficient way of accessing the literature, taking it in turns to research a particular topic. And when you do so, don't go straight for *Medline*, unless you hold a black belt in search strategies. There are many good sources of pre-digested evidence and summaries available to assist you, ranging from the gold standards of the *Cochrane Database of Systematic Reviews* and *Clinical Evidence*, to review articles in some of the better 'glossies' such as *Practitioner* and *Update*.

Above all, expand your experience. General practice is about people, their thoughts, feelings, cultures and relationships. This you don't get from medical textbooks, but you might from a film, a novel or a play. Use these sources and your understanding of, and communication with, patients will be greatly enhanced.

The books and websites we have mentioned in the guide are mainly for reference. This chapter summarises our recommended reading, but the list is by no means exclusive and we would love to hear your suggestions for inclusion in future editions.

What to read

The nature of general practice

Fry J (1983) *The Future General Practitioner*. Royal College of General Practitioners, London.

Fry J (1999) *Common Diseases, their Nature, Incidence and Care (5e)*. Librapharm/Petroc Press, Newbury.

Heath I (1995) *The Mystery of General Practice*. Nuffield Provincial Hospitals Trust, London.

Helman C (1990) *Culture, Health and Illness*. Butterworth-Heinemann, Oxford.

Lane K (1992) *The Longest Art*. Royal College of General Practitioners, London.

Pringle M (1998) *Core Values in Primary Care.* BMJ Books, London.

Qureshi B (1998) *Transcultural Medicine: dealing with patients from different cultures.* Librapharm/Petroc Press, Newbury.

Rakel R (2002) *Textbook of Family Practice (6e).* WB Saunders, Philadelphia.

Rosenthal J, Naish J and Lloyd M (1994) *The Trainee's Companion to General Practice.* Churchill Livingstone, London.

Simon C, Everitt H, Birtwisle J and Stevenson B (2002) *The Oxford Handbook of General Practice.* Oxford University Press, Oxford.

The consultation

Balint M (1957) *The Doctor, his Patient and the Illness.* Pitman Medical, London.

Bendix T (1982) *The Anxious Patient.* Churchill Livingstone, Edinburgh.

Berne E (1966) *Games People Play.* Andre Deutsch, London.

Neighbour RH (1987) *The Inner Consultation.* MTP Press, Lancaster.

Pendleton D, Schofield T, Tate P *et al.* (1984) *The Consultation: an approach to learning and teaching.* Oxford University Press, Oxford.

Silverman J, Kurtz S and Draper J (1998) *Skills for Communicating with Patients.* Radcliffe Medical Press, Oxford.

Tate P (1997) *The Doctor's Communication Handbook.* Radcliffe Medical Press, Oxford.

Psychosocial disease in general practice

Armstrong E (1995) *Mental Health Issues in Primary Care: a practical guide.* Palgrave Macmillan, Basingstoke.

Banks (1994) *Drug Misuse: a practical handbook for the GP*. Blackwell Scientific, London.

Craig T and Davies T (1998) *ABC of Mental Health*. BMJ Books, London.

DOH (1999) *Drug Misuse and Dependence: guidelines on clinical management*. The Stationery Office, London.

Egan G (1994) *The Skilled Helper (5e)*. Brooks/Cole Publishing, California.

Gelder M, Gath D, Mayou R and Cowen P (1996) *Oxford Textbook of Psychiatry (3e)*. Oxford University Press, Oxford.

Keithley J and Marsh G (1995) *Counseling in Primary Health Care*. Oxford University Press, Oxford.

Kendrick T, Tylee A and Freeling P (1996) *The Prevention of Mental Illness in Primary Care*. Cambridge University Press, Cambridge.

Nelson Jones R (1997) *Practical Counselling and Helping Skills*. Cassell, London.

Ogden J (1996) *Health Psychology: a textbook*. Open University, Buckingham.

Paton A (1994) *ABC of Alcohol (3e)*. BMJ Books, London.

Salinsky J and Sackin P (2002) *What Are You Feeling, Doctor?* Radcliffe Medical Press, Oxford.

Skinner R and Cleese J (1993) *Families and How to Survive Them*. Random House, UK.

Undifferentiated and trivial problems in general practice

Fry J and Sandler G (1998) *Common Diseases, their Nature, Incidence and Care (5e)*. Librapharm/Petroc Press, Newbury.

Hopcroft K and Forte V (1999) *Symptom Sorter*. Radcliffe Medical Press, Oxford.

Johnson G, Hill-Smith I and Ellis C (1999) *The Minor Illness Manual*. Radcliffe Medical Press, Oxford.

Knot A and Polmear A (1999) *Practical General Practice.* Butterworth-Heinemann, Oxford.

Stearn M (1998) *Embarrassing Problems.* Health Press, Oxford.

Emergencies in general practice

Brown A (2002) *Accident and Emergency Diagnosis and Management (4e).* Arnold Press, London.

Dwight O and Collier J (eds) (2001) *Guidelines for the Management of Common Medical Emergencies in General Practice.* National Patients Access Team, London.

Harrington R, Hope S, Watts J and Lawrence N (1996) *Handbook of Emergencies in General Practice (2e).* Oxford University Press, Oxford.

Mehta DK (ed) *British National Formulary.* BMA and the Royal Pharmaceutical Society of Great Britain, London.

General medical problems and the management of chronic disease

Barton S (ed) (2002) *Clinical Evidence.* BMJ Publishing Group, London.

Clark M and Kumar P (2002) *Clinical Medicine (5e).* WB Saunders, Philadelphia.

Hasler J (1996) *The Management of Chronic Disease.* Oxford University Press, Oxford.

Longmore JM, Longmore M, Torok E and Wilkinson I (2001) *Oxford Handbook of Clinical Medicine.* Oxford University Press Inc. USA.

McWhinney I (1997) *A Textbook of Family Medicine.* Oxford University Press, Oxford.

Ear, nose and throat

Browning GG (1994) *Updated ENT (3e)*. Butterworth-Heinemann, Oxford.

Ludman H (1997) *ABC of Otolaryngology*. BMJ Books, London.

Rheumatology and orthopaedics

Carr A and Harnden A (1995) *Orthopaedics in Primary Care*. Butterworth-Heinmann, Oxford.

Hutson MA (1996) *Sports Injuries: recognition and management (2e)*. Oxford University Press, Oxford.

Silver T (2001) *Joint and Soft Tissue Injection (3e)*. Radcliffe Medical Press, Oxford.

Snaith M (1999) *ABC of Rheumatology (2e)*. BMJ Books, London.

Eye problems

Finlay RD and Payne PAG (1997) *The Eye in General Practice (10e)*. Butterworth-Heinemann, Oxford.

Khaw PT (1999) *ABC of Eyes*. BMJ Books, London.

Okhravi N (1997) *Manual of Primary Eye Care*. Butterworth-Heinemann, Oxford.

Women's health

Anthony J and Kaye P (2001) *Notes for the DRCOG (4e)*. Churchill Livingstone, Oxford.

Guillebaud J (1997) *The Pill and Other Forms of Hormonal Contraception*. Oxford Paperbacks, Oxford.

Guillebaud J (1999) *Contraception: your questions answered.* Churchill Livingstone, Oxford.

McPherson A and Waller D (1997) *Women's Health (4e).* Oxford University Press, Oxford.

The care of babies and children

Goldman A (1994) *Care of the Dying Child.* Oxford University Press, Oxford.

Hall D, Hill P and Ellman D (1994) *The Child Surveillance Handbook.* Radcliffe Medical Press, Oxford.

Hall D (1996) *Health for all Children.* Oxford University Press, Oxford.

Hull D and Johnston D (1993) *Essential Paediatrics.* Churchill Livingstone, Edinburgh.

Illingworth R (1991) *The Normal Child.* Churchill Livingstone, Edinburgh.

Modell M, Mughal Z and Boyd R (1996) *Paediatric Problems in General Practice.* Oxford University Press, Oxford.

Valman H (1993) *ABC of One to Seven.* BMJ Books, London.

Sexual medicine

Adler M (1998) *ABC of AIDS (5e).* BMJ Books, London.

Adler M (1998) *ABC of Sexually Transmitted Disease (5e).* BMJ Books, London.

Bancroft J (1989) *Human Sexuality and its Problems (2e)* Churchill Livingstone, Edinburgh.

Carter Y, Moss C and Weyman A (1997) *RCGP Handbook of Sexual Health in Primary Care.* Royal College of General Practitioners, London.

Skrine R (1997) *Blocks and Freedoms in Sexual Life: a handbook of psychosexual medicine.* Radcliffe Medical Press, Oxford.

Skin problems

Buxton P (1998) *ABC of Dermatology (3e)*. BMJ Books, London.

Du Vivier A (2002) *Atlas of Clinical Dermatology (3e)*. Churchill Livingstone, Edinburgh.

Hunter J, Savin J and Dahl M (1994) *Clinical Dermatology*. Blackwell, Oxford.

Kneebone R and Schofield J (1998) *Minor Surgery and Skin Lesions, CD-ROM*. Royal College of General Practitioners, London.

Stuart Brown J (2001) *Minor Surgery: a text and atlas (3e)*. Arnold, London.

Care of the elderly

Coni N, Davison W and Webster S (1992*) Ageing: the facts (2e)*. Oxford University Press, Oxford.

Department of Health (2002) *National Service Framework for Elderly Care*. DoH, London.

Grimsley Evans J and Franklin William T (1992) *Oxford Textbook of Geriatric Medicine*. Oxford University Press, Oxford.

Idris Williams E (1995) *Caring for Older People in the Community*. Radcliffe Medical Press, Oxford.

Sidell M (1995) *Health in Old Age: myth, mystery and management*. Oxford University Press, Oxford.

Terminal care and bereavement

Doyle D (1994) *Domiciliary Palliative Care: a handbook for family doctors and community nurses*. Oxford University Press, Oxford.

Kubler-Ross E (1973) *On Death and Dying*. Routlege, London.

Parkes CM (1998) *Bereavement: studies of grief in adult life*. Penguin, London.

Preventive medicine and immunisation

Austoker J (1995) *Cancer Prevention in Primary Care*. BMJ Books, London.

Department of Health (1996) *Immunisation against Infectious Disease*. The Stationery Office, London.

Fowler G, Muir Gray J and Anderson P (1993) *Prevention in General Practice*. Oxford University Press, Oxford.

Naidoo J and Willis J (1994) *Health Promotion: foundations for practice*. Balliere Tindall, London.

Walker E, Williams G and Raeside F (1997) *ABC of Health Travel*. BMJ Books, London.

Prescribing

See Topic 18, p. 103.

Management and finance in general practice

Belbin RM (1981) *Management Teams: why they succeed or fail*. Heinemann Professional Publishing, Oxford.

Bogle I (2002) *Succeeding as a General Practitioner: the experts share their secrets*. Health Press, Oxford.

Bogle I, Chisholm J and Ellis N (1997) *Making Sense of the Red Book*. Radcliffe Medical Press, Oxford.

Chisholm J, Ellis N and Lawrence-Parr C (1998) *General Practice Employment Handbook*. Radcliffe Medical Press, Oxford.

Dean J (2000) *Making Sense of Practice Finance*. Radcliffe Medical Press, Oxford.

Elwyn G, Greenhalgh T and Macfarlane F (2001) *Groups: a guide to small group work in healthcare, management, education and research*. Radcliffe Medical Press, Oxford.

Irvine S and Haman H (1997) *Making Sense of Personnel Management*. Radcliffe Medical Press, Oxford.

Jay A (1976) *How to Run a Meeting*. Booklet to accompany the film '*Meetings, Bloody Meetings*'. Video Arts, London.

Pringle M (1993) *Change and Teamwork in Primary Care*. BMJ Books, London.

Pritchard P and Pritchard J (1992) *Developing Teamwork in Primary Health Care*. Oxford Medical Publications, Oxford.

The organisation of healthcare

Boyd R (1996) *What is the Future for a Primary Care-led NHS?* Radcliffe Medical Press, Oxford.

Audit, quality and clinical governance

Greenhalgh T (1997) *How to Read a Paper*. BMJ Books, London.

Guyatt G and Drummond R (2002) *Users' Guides to the Medical Literature*. AMA Press, Chicago.

Mulligan J (1988) *The Personal Management Handbook: how to make the most of your potential*. Sphere, London.

Rughani A (2000) *The GP's Guide to Personal Development Plans*. Radcliffe Medical Press, Oxford.

Ethics, probity and the law

Beauchamp T and Childress J (2001) *Principles of Biomedical Ethics (5e)*. Oxford University Press, Oxford.

Essex B (1994) *Doctors, Dilemmas, Decisions*. BMJ Books, London.

General Medical Council (2001) *Good Medical Practice (3e)*. GMC, London.

Gillon R (1986) *Philosophical Medical Ethics*. John Wiley and Sons, Chichester.

Pickersgill D (1992) *The Law and General Practice*. Radcliffe Medical Press, Oxford.

Royal College of General Practitioners and the General Practitioner Committee of the BMA (2002) *Good Medical Practice for General Practitioners*. RCGP, London.

Toon P (1999) *Towards a Philosophy of General Practice: a study of the virtuous practitioner*. Occasional Paper No. 78. Royal College of General Practitioners, London.

Useful websites

Searching the internet for information has become very easy, thanks to the National electronic Library for Health (NeLH). The NeLH is a national web-based information resource for the NHS providing access to a range of high quality information resources. The library is available 24 hours a day and can be accessed free of charge by anyone. Some of the licensed resources, such as the *Cochrane Library*, may only be available via the NHS net or on registering for a password. Sites available through the NeLH incude: Bandolier, British National Formulary, the *Cochrane Library*, Medline, PubMed, National Institute for Clinical Excellence and Prodigy. There are also professional portals and virtual branch libraries for the various specialties. Why not go on line and have a look at www.nelh.nhs.uk.

Other sites that will also be of some interest include:

British Medical Association	www.bma.org.uk
General Medical Council	www.gmc.org.uk
Royal College of General Practitioners	www.rcgp.org.uk
JCPTGP	www.jcptgp.org.uk
Department of Health	www.doh.gov.uk
National Health Service	www.nhs.uk

Index